THE SECRET OF CHINESE PULSE DIAGNOSIS

THE SECRET OF Chinese Pulse Diagnosis

Bob Flaws

BLUE POPPY PRESS

Published by:

BLUE POPPY PRESS, INC.
1775 LINDEN AVE.
BOULDER, CO 80304

FIRST EDITION, SEPTEMBER 1995

ISBN 0-936185-67-8 LC #95-80457

COMP Designation: Original work and functionally translated compilation using a standard translational terminology.

Printed at Hignell Printing Limited, Winnipeg, Manitoba, Canada on acid free, elementally chlorine free paper.

Cover art by Jeff Fuller, Crescent Moon

The cover picture is of the divine doctor, Qi Bo. It has been lent to us by the kind permission of Signor L. Paroli of GMT 2000, Laveno, Italy, publisher of the Italian Journal, *Yi Dao.*

10 9 8 7 6 5 4 3 2

Preface

The first person with whom I studied Chinese medicine instilled in me a high regard for the pulse. The things he was able to tell people after feeling their pulses for fifteen minutes seemed like magic to me. Some time later, I studied pulse diagnosis in Tibetan medicine with various lama-doctors. There, too, pulse reading seemed to endow its practitioners with almost magical abilities of diagnosis and prognosis. Therefore, I believe I was fortunate to come across teachers who emphasized the value of pulse examination.

Nevertheless, it took me years to learn how to read the pulse. The years this required were not because of any inherent difficulty in feeling and interpreting the pulse, but were due to my own laziness and stubborn refusal to master the basics of this art. While I searched for advanced and abstruse pulse lore, I was never diligent enough to memorize all the basic facts of this discipline. In other words, I tried to jump high up in the sky without first laying an adequate foundation. As a teacher of Traditional Chinese Medicine, it is my experience that all too many of my fellow Western practitioners make the same mistake.

The impetus for writing this book is, therefore, based on my own personal experience with the pulse. It is my attempt to share with my fellow practitioners a central insight which has meant the difference between a mediocre ability to read the pulse and an ability which most of my peers consider advanced. As the reader will see, this advanced ability, to the degree that it exists, exists because of finally mastering the basics.

Because I wish the reader to concentrate on a few key points which must then be memorized to perfection, I have not tried to write an exhaustive or encyclopedic book on the pulse. Rather, this book is meant to complement and extend other books on Chinese diagnosis and pulse examination which already exist in English. This is a deliberately small book.

The terminology in this book is based on Nigel Wiseman's *Glossary of Chinese Medical Terms and Acupuncture Points*, Paradigm Publications, Brookline, MA, 1990. This book is a compilation of information taken from a variety of Chinese and English language sources. A bibliography of those sources is appended at the end of this book.

During my first Tibetan language lesson, my teacher began by having me spell out the Tibetan word "easy". At the time, it was explained to me that this was to ensure a good omen at the beginning. Looking back, I see it as a reminder that if we begin a task with the preconception that it is hard, we are less likely to persevere to the point of mastery. However, if we begin with the idea that something is easy, then we do not have to constantly fight our own preconceived notions to the contrary. I believe that too many students in the West believe that Chinese pulse examination is difficult to learn and that it takes years and years to master. Thinking thus, many of us Westerners put off mastering the basic information to the degree that information can be put into practical use in the clinic. Hence the pulse is never really mastered.

Therefore, this book has been written with one main intention in mind: to put forward the notion that Chinese pulse examination is easy *if one knows the secret*. That secret is mastering the basics.

Bob Flaws
May 10, 1995

Contents

1
Introduction

This book is a basic introduction to pulse examination as it is used in Traditional Chinese Medicine or TCM. Although in Chinese, TCM is simply referred to as *zhong yi* or Chinese medicine, I do regard what is usually called TCM in the West as a particular style of Chinese medicine. Many of the adherents of this style would simply say that TCM encompasses all that has been found to be worthwhile and clinically valid over the 2000 years of recorded Chinese medical history and that is why it is simply called Chinese medicine. Be that as it may, here in the West, there are a number of styles of Oriental medicine currently being taught and practiced. Therefore, I think it useful to distinguish this style for what it is. Hence, before attempting to understand the role and practice of pulse examination within this style, I believe it is important to understand something about this style in general.

TCM as a Style

The hallmark of TCM as a style of Chinese medicine is its emphasis on treatment based on pattern discrimination (*bian zheng lun zhi*). This means that, although TCM practitioners first make a disease diagnosis (*bian bing*), treatment is based more on the pattern discrimination than on that disease diagnosis. In other words, the overall guiding treatment principles for the case at hand are based on the pattern discrimination, not on the disease diagnosis. It is these principles which guide the selection of the Chinese medicinal formula or main acupuncture points. Once these main principles are stated and a basic treatment protocol is erected based on these principles, medicinals or acupuncture points are then added to the base protocol depending on their empirical efficacy for the particular disease under treatment.

For instance, a patient may be suffering from headache. In TCM, headache (*tou tong*) is a disease category. If the patient also says that her headache comes at the end of every menstruation, is worse at night or when fatigued, tends to be generalized, typically lasts until she goes to bed but is usually gone when she wakes the next morning, and if her facial complexion is a sallow yellow, she has palpitations or dizziness, lack of warmth in her four limbs, a scanty appetite, loose stools with her period, pale nails, a pale tongue, and a fine and weak or relaxed pulse, her TCM pattern discrimination is one of blood vacuity due to spleen vacuity. In that case, the main treatment principles are to fortify the spleen and nourish the blood. The guiding formula in that case might be either *Ba Zhen Tang* (Eight Pearls Decoction) or *Gui Pi Tang* (Restore the Spleen Decoction) depending upon the exact signs and symptoms. If *Gui Pi Tang* were chosen, then Radix Ligustici Wallichii (*Chuan Xiong*) might be added to specifically upbear blood to nourish the sea of marrow and therefore address the specific complaint of headache.

If treated by acupuncture, the basic formula might consist of *Zu San Li* (St 36), *San Yin Jiao* (Sp 6), *Pi Shu* (Bl 20), and *Ge Shu* (Bl 17). The first three points all fortify the spleen, remembering that it is the spleen which is the root of latter heaven or postnatal qi and blood engenderment and transformation. *Ge Shu* is the *hui* or so-called reunion point of the blood. It specifically acts to nourish the blood. If the major complaint or disease were palpitations, then *Shen Men* (Ht 7) might be added to this basic formula. However, because the disease under treatment is headache, *Bai Hui* (GV 20) might be added with moxibustion in order to upbear yang qi, based on the premise that it is the qi which moves the blood and that the blood follows the qi.

It is said in TCM:

> *Yi bing tong zhi*
> *Tong bing yi zhi*
> One disease, different treatments;
> Different diseases, one treatment.

This means that any disease may present a number of different patterns. In the case of headache, there are wind cold external invasion pattern headaches, liver yang hyperactive above pattern headaches, phlegm dampness obstructing the clear portals pattern headaches, blood vacuity pattern headaches, and essence insufficiency pattern headaches, to name the most common ones. Although two patients may each suffer from headache, if their TCM pattern discrimination is different, they will receive a different treatment. Another two patients may present with two completely different diseases. One may be suffering from headache and the other from insomnia and yet, as long as they present the same overall TCM pattern, their treatment may be essentially the same.

Therefore, in TCM, a correct pattern discrimination is vitally important. It is the guide and foundation to successful, individualized treatment. When treatment is given on the basis of a correct TCM pattern discrimination, it restores balance without iatrogenesis or side effects. In addition, a TCM pattern discrimination contains within itself an explanation of why the person is manifesting the signs and symptoms they do. Each pattern is the result of certain disease causes (*bing yin*) and disease mechanisms (*bing ji*). If one understands those disease causes and mechanisms, then one can take steps to alter or abolish them. One can change their diet and lifestyle accordingly and even change deleterious mental/emotional habits. Thus a TCM pattern discrimination is both enlightening and empowering in a way that a simple disease diagnosis typically is not. Hence, TCM pattern discriminations are the means by which practitioners of Chinese medicine can follow the injunctions in the *Nei Jing (Inner Classic)* to emphasize prevention over mere remedial treatment.

How Patterns Are Discriminated

TCM patterns are discriminated by means of the four examinations (*si zhen*). These are visual examination (*wang zhen*), inquiry (*wen zhen*), listening and smelling examination (*wen zhen*), and palpation (*qie zhen*). It is by means of the combination of these four methods of examination (*si zhen he can*) that a TCM pattern is identified. However, most modern TCM clinical manuals describe this combined summation and analysis in terms of main symptoms (*zhu zheng*), examination of the tongue (*she zhen*), and pulse examination (*mai zhen*). In other words, in clinical practice, patterns are based on three broad groups of information: 1) signs and symptoms, 2) tongue examination, and 3) pulse examination. It is the comparison and corroboration of these three groups of information which differentiate one pattern from another, and it is extremely important that no one sign or symptom means anything except in relationship to all other signs and symptoms gathered by the four examinations.

For instance, the pattern of spleen qi vacuity and spleen yang vacuity have many of the same signs and symptoms. In both patterns there are scanty appetite, loose stools, abdominal distention, fatigue, lack of strength, and a pale tongue with a thin, white coating. However, in the case of spleen yang vacuity there are also chilling of the limbs, a cold body, and a slow pulse. But this does not mean that chilled limbs are always a symptom of yang vacuity. There may be chilled limbs due to liver depression/qi stagnation. In this case, the four chilled limbs are referred to as the four counterflows because yang qi is depressed internally and cannot flow uninhibitedly out to the extremities. One knows this because the tongue in this case is a dark reddish and may have a yellowish coating, while the pulse is wiry and rapid, not slow.

Thus it is vitally important to keep in mind that no one sign or symptom always means any one thing. It only means something when taken in consideration of all other signs and symptoms, including the tongue and pulse examinations.

The TCM Methodology

This basic TCM methodology of moving from a major complaint to the patient's individual signs and symptoms, tongue, and pulse, thus constituting the pattern discrimination, thence to the statement of treatment principles, and only then to the selection of a guiding formula or protocol and its individualized modifications is exemplified in the organization of most modern Chinese TCM clinical manuals. In such clinical handbooks, information is typically given under the following headings and in the following order:

Disease name:
Treatment based on pattern discrimination:
Pattern name:
Main symptoms:
Tongue & coating:
Pulse images:
Treatment principles:
Formula:
Additions & subtractions based on symptoms:

Just as most Chinese clinical manuals and textbooks are organized in this manner, it is important that clinicians follow this methodology or progression when making a pattern discrimination and then erecting a treatment plan. This is a very step by step methodology, and if one omits a step, then the whole process may go awry. It is especially important to write down the TCM pattern discrimination and the treatment principles before writing down the names of Chinese medicinal formulas or acupuncture points. I have explained this process at greater length in both my *Sticking to the Point: A Rational Methodology for the Step by Step Formulation & Administration of a TCM Acupuncture Treatment* and *How to Write a TCM Herbal Formula.*

The Importance of Pulse Examination

As seen above, pulse examination is one of the main methods of establishing a TCM pattern discrimination. Pulse examination in modern TCM primarily means the feeling of the pulse of the radial arteries at the styloid processes of both wrists. This is commonly called the *cun kou* or inch opening. It is believed by practitioners of Chinese medicine that the pulses felt here can be read as a simulacrum of the flow of qi, blood, and body fluids of the entire body. The first chapter of the *Nan Jing (Classic of Difficulties)* opens with the following question:

> All the twelve channels have [sections where the] movement [in these] vessels [can be felt]. Still, one selects only the *cun kou* in order to determine whether the five viscera and six bowels [harbor a] pattern of death or life, of good or evil auspices. What does that mean?[1]

The answer of why one can determine the health and disease of the entire body by feeling the pulses at the *cun kou* on the wrists that the *Nan Jing* gives is this:

> The *cun kou* constitutes the great meeting point of the [contents passing through] the vessels. It is the [section of] the hand *tai yin* [channel where the] movement [in that] vessel [can be felt]. When a [normal] person exhales once, [the contents of] the vessels proceed 3 inches. When [a normal person] inhales once, [the contents of] the vessels proceed [another] 3 inches. Exhaling and inhaling [constitute one] breathing [period]. During this period, [the contents of] the vessels proceed 6 inches. A person, in the course of one day and one night, breathes altogether 13,500 times. [During that time, the contents of] the vessels proceed through 50 passages. [That is,] they circulate through the body [in the period needed by] the [clepsydra's] dripping water to move down by 100 markings. The constructive and defensive [qi] proceed through 25 passages [during a] yang [period], and they proceed through 25 passages [during a] yin [period]. This constitutes one cycle. Because [the contents of the vessels] meet again, after 50 passages, with the *cun kou*, [this section] is the beginning and the end of [movement of the contents of the vessels through the body's] five viscera and six bowels. Hence, the pattern [of death or life, good or evil auspices harbored by the body's five viscera and six bowels] may be obtained from the *cun kou*.[2]

Whether or how one chooses to accept this explanation aside, it is a fact that practitioners of Chinese medicine have been diagnosing and treating patients on the basis of pulse examination carried out at the inch opening

---

1 *Nan Ching (The Classic of Difficulties)*, trans. by Paul U. Unschuld, University of California Press, Berkeley, CA, 1986, p. 65. Some words have been changed to conform to Nigel Wiseman's terminology.

2 *Ibid.*, p. 65-66

for at least 2000 years. On the other hand, most Western students of TCM find pulse examination very confusing and difficult to master. It seems somehow very mystical and arcane. Although most Western practitioners express a strong belief and interest in pulse examination, few, I think, feel very confident of their abilities in this domain.

This Western ambivalence toward and pervasive lack of mastery of pulse examination is, I believe, exacerbated by a somewhat similar attitude toward pulse examination current in the Peoples' Republic of China at least in the 1980s. When I was a student in China during that time, the importance of pulse examination was deliberately played down by many of my teachers and clinical preceptors. Based on conversations, it seems they felt that pulse examination was hard to validate by Western anatomy and physiology and, therefore, was a bit of an embarrassment to people who were desperately trying to become modern and scientific. At that time, I never had a teacher tell me a pulse was anything other than wiry, slippery, fast, slow, floating, deep, or fine. One of my teachers only took the pulse with two fingers and never expressed her readings in terms of the three basic positions of the pulse. When queried about this, she said that it is scientifically impossible for the pulse to have different qualities or images in different positions. *Ergo*, one does not have to worry about positions.

What I mean to say is that, although pulse examination comprises at least one third of the diagnostic criteria for making a TCM pattern discrimination, many modern Chinese teachers and the majority of the modern Chinese TCM literature of which I am aware, tend not to be very sophisticated in their explanation and use of pulse examination. Rather, it seems that many modern Chinese TCM practitioners relegate pulse examination to a minor, confirmatory role. While Western practitioners believe that pulse examination is mystical, and therefore difficult to learn, many modern Chinese practitioners believe it is mystical, and therefore not worth learning.

However, this is not my experience. I believe that mastery of pulse examination is vitally important for making a correct TCM pattern discrimination. And I believe that pulse examination is, perhaps, even more important for Western practitioners than for our Chinese counterparts. This is because it is my experience that our patients are sick in more complex ways than many Chinese patients. In China, most young practitioners do not go into private practice working in isolation from senior practitioners with lifetimes of experience. It is my experience that young practitioners in China are given relatively simple cases to treat, and, should they come across a complicated, difficult case, they can always ask a senior practitioner to help parse out the pattern discrimination. Western practitioners, on the other hand, tend to go immediately into private practice, and that after insufficient clinical education as an undergraduate. Typically, there is no one else in the clinic to ask about a difficult case. In addition, we as Western practitioners tend to see a disproportionate number of difficult cases which are either not self-limiting or have not been successfully treated by modern Western medicine and often other types of alternative medicine as well. This is because, here in the West, we are so often practitioners of last resort. Further, because of the modern Western diet, the adverse effects of certain modern Western medical treatments, the ill effects of pollution, and the pervasive stress of our modern society, most of our patients suffer from complex, chronic conditions which frequently and I might even say typically do not display the nice, neat, simple patterns contained in beginners' TCM textbooks.

In my experience, all too often, our patients present, not with one textbook pattern or another, but with a combination of three, four, or even five patterns. When the disease mechanisms at work in such complex patterns interact with each other, they produce complicated mixtures of signs and symptoms, including complicated and sometimes even seemingly contrary pulse images. Thus it is also my experience that if one wants to parse out such complicated patterns, one must be able to feel more than just the several pulse images enumerated above. In addition, one must also understand how each pulse is created and the secondary and tertiary meanings of all of the pulse images. In other words, it is my experience that a simplistic approach to pulse examination is not sufficient for the practice of TCM in the West.

The Obstacles to Mastering the Pulse

The good news is that pulse examination is not that difficult to master. In my experience, there is a trick that makes pulse examination actually quite easy and straightforward. However, before revealing that secret, I would like to quote Manfred Porkert from *The Essentials of Chinese Diagnostics* on what he calls "three kinds of obstacles to mastering pulse diagnosis:"[3]

1. Inadequate endowment
2. Wrong intellectual perspective
3. Inapt pedagological approach

Manfred Porkert describes inadequate natural endowment under two subheadings: 1) inadequate physical endowment (*i.e.*, lack of sufficient sensitivity in the fingertips and the capability to concentrate) and 2) inadequate intellectual gifts (*i.e.*, inability to distinguish, coordinate, and synthesize the observed data). In terms of this first obstacle to mastering Chinese pulse examination, it is up to the Deans of Admission and Academic Deans at Western schools and colleges of acupuncture and Oriental medicine to ensure that all students enrolled at such schools are endowed with these capabilities.

By "wrong intellectual perspective," Porkert is referring to preconceived notions regarding Chinese pulse examination by Western health care practitioners who are often skeptical about it. If one refuses to believe that one can diagnose health and disease by feeling the pulse of the radial arteries at the wrists, then of course, one will not seriously study this art with an open mind and will not plumb its depths. This is not usually a problem at most Western schools of acupuncture and Oriental medicine. Students at such schools typically enter with a willingness to study and consider as at least provisionally true the basic theories and practices of Chinese medicine.

---

[3] Porkert, Manfred, *The Essentials of Chinese Diagnostics*, Chinese Medicine Publications, Ltd., Zurich, Switzerland, 1983, p. 193

However, it is the last obstacle—an inapt pedagological approach—which Porkert says is responsible for most failures in mastering Chinese pulse examination. In fact, it is Porkert's opinion that:

> Most of the failures in mastering pulse diagnosis—I should say at least 80 percent—are due to this formidable obstacle, or to approaching it too lightly.[4]

According to Porkert, Chinese pulse examination is a skill. However, it is an essentially intellectual skill. He goes on to say that in the acquisition of any skill, the gathering of certain intellectual information *must* precede physical training. This means that intellectual data must be presented before physical instruction and that it is that intellectual data which actually constitutes the indispensable basis for the effective acquisition, assimilation, and integration of physical experience. In other words and in terms of Chinese pulse examination, unless one has learned all pertinent TCM theory and the intellectual, *i.e.*, verbal, descriptions of all the major pulse images, one cannot feel and interpret the pulses correctly.

To exemplify this point, several years ago, in going back through my case records, I noticed that I had often written down that this or that patient's pulse was fine and floating. At the time, I had just finished reviewing the textbook definitions of the 28 pulses and these were fresh in my mind. I immediately recognized that what I had described as a fine and floating pulse is the soggy (*ru*) or soft (*ruan*) pulse. I had been feeling fine and floating pulses for years. However, until I realized that a fine and floating pulse is a soggy pulse, I was not able to make the diagnoses that go with a soggy or soft pulse. My fingers were not suddenly feeling anything physically different. My new-found ability to feel the soggy pulse was entirely an intellectual capability, a verbal epiphany, not a physical one.

---

[4] *Ibid.*, p. 195

The Secret of Chinese Pulse Examination

In my experience, the secret of Chinese pulse examination is exactly this: *One cannot feel a pulse image unless one can consciously and accurately state the standard, textbook definition of that pulse image.* If one does not know that the soggy pulse is floating and fine, one cannot write down that diagnosis even though one may be able to feel that the pulse is floating and fine. Therefore, I wholeheartedly agree with Porkert when he says:

> Applied to the training and mastery of pulse diagnosis...the problem is not that the students cannot feel what must be felt, but that they usually are at a loss to describe, hence to assimilate, to permanently learn and keep what they have physically perceived... This, precisely, is the critical issue: there is no point in attempting practical training in pulse diagnosis *unless all pertinent theory and, more important, the complete iconography of the pulse has previously been absorbed intellectually.* In other words, no student of pulse diagnosis should attempt practical training unless he has not only memorized, but understood by frequent rehearsal, every single term and technical relationship instrumental to Chinese pulse diagnosis... Only on this condition will he be able to immediately describe and express with precision and stringency what he feels when actually putting his fingers on a patient's arms. And only on this premise will he be able to recall, reflect and communicate to his colleagues what he feels.[5]

Porkert goes on to state:

> If this essential condition has been met, practical mastery of pulse diagnosis in normal medical practice is—at worst—a question of several months; with proper guidance it should take only weeks to gauge, correct and refine one's sensitivity so that the error rate drops to insignificance within one month. If, on the contrary, this warning is ignored, even with the best intentions, a student may not master quite basic notions even with years of trying... Trying to make sense of the subtle differences felt at the pulse sites without the most strict reference and conscientious attention to the intellectual tools prepared *for this very purpose* in the course of almost 2000 years is like attempting to interpret an EKG while spurning all

[5] *Ibid.*, p. 196

> knowledge of what is taught about this technique in medical colleges by physics, physiology and clinical medicine.[6]

I have to admit that this is exactly the case with me and my experience of Chinese pulse examination. I first read Porkert's book in 1983 when it was first published in English. At the time, I remember reading the above passages. I did not just read them, I even underlined them. However, I did not actually take the trouble to memorize the exact Chinese definitions of all the major pulse images until several years ago. Although I was able to feel the slow and fast, deep and floating, slippery, wiry, and fine pulses, as long as I could not say either out loud or to myself the word for word definitions of the other 20 or more pulses, I could not feel them in clinical practice. Once I realized this fact and went back and memorized these definitions, I was immediately able to feel all the major pulses *as long as I kept these definitions currently in mind.* In addition, I have taught this approach to several groups of Western students and, within two days, they were immediately able to feel and consciously identify twice as many pulses as they had been previously able.

In other words, this method works. I know it works because it works for me. I also know it works because I have seen it work for others as well. Having studied several Oriental arts in my life, it is my experience that mastery comes from mastering the basics. Unless there is a solid foundation, one cannot build high into the sky. Beginners think that masters have some special secrets to which they are not yet privy, but that is rarely the case. Mastery always means mastery of the basics. Unfortunately, all too often it is human nature to be impatient with the basics and to try to jump to some seemingly higher, more exciting plane. In terms of Chinese pulse examination, mastery of the basics primarily means the memorization of the definitions of the major pulse images or what Manfred Porkert calls the iconography of the pulse.

This is not a big book on the pulse. Certainly there is more that can be said about Chinese pulse examination. However, it is my heart-felt plea that

---

6 *Ibid.*, p. 196

Western students of acupuncture and Oriental medicine not just read this book but take the time to memorize the factual material it contains. At the very least, if you want to be able to feel the main 27-29 pulse images, *you must memorize their definitions*. As Manfred Porkert points out:

> Chinese pulse diagnosis does not presuppose any exceptional, little known, paranormal endowment or ability in the person applying it. All that is required is a solid grounding in its coherent theory and a trained and well-kept hand.[7]

For many modern Western students, memorization is a dirty word. It seems so boring and prosaic. It seems to lack mystery and imagination. But believe me, if you want to be able to do Chinese pulse examination, just do it.

---

7 *Ibid.*, p. 197

2
The Divisions of the Pulse at the Inch Opening & Their Correspondences

Contemporary TCM primarily makes use of the radial artery pulse at the styloid processes on both wrists. As mentioned above, this is called the *cun kou* or inch opening. It is believed that one can feel a simulacrum of the qi, blood, and body fluids of the entire body at this anatomical position. This basic anatomical location is divided both longitudinally from distal to proximal and in terms of depth, from superficial to deep. Longitudinally, the inch opening is divided into three basic divisions. Nigel Wiseman refers to these as:

Cun, inch
Guan, bar
Chi, cubit

If the practitioner takes the patient's right pulse with their left hand, the *guan* or bar pulse (also called the barrier or gate pulse) is felt directly under the practitioner's middle finger when that is allowed to rest on the patient's styloid process. The *cun* or inch pulse is then felt by the practitioner's index finger which is resting in the space between the styloid process and the base of the thenar eminence. The cubit or *chi* pulse is found directly under the practitioner's ring finger, immediately proximal to their middle finger resting on the patient's styloid process. Typically, when all three of these positions are spoken of, they are named from distal to proximal: inch, bar, cubit, *cun, guan, chi*.

The names of these positions are derived from the fact that the *chi* or cubit pulse is located one *chi* or foot from the ventral crease of the elbow joint.

The names of these positions are derived from the fact that the *chi* or cubit pulse is located one *chi* or foot from the ventral crease of the elbow joint. The *cun* or inch pulse is located in the one inch wide space between the styloid process and the base of the thenar eminence. The styloid process then sticks up like a bar or barrier between these two positions, and hence the name *guan*, bar, barrier, or gate.

The identification of these three positions goes back to at least the *Nan Jing (Classic of Difficulties)* or around the 2nd century CE. The second chapter of that classic states:

> The cubit and inch [section] is the great important meeting-point of the [movements in the] vessels. [The distance] from the bar to the cubit [marsh in the elbow, *i.e.*, the acupuncture point *Chi Ze*, Lu 5] represents the foot interior [section]... [The distance] from the bar to the fish line [*i.e.*, the base of the thenar eminence] represents the inch interior [section]... Hence, [one] inch is separated [from the entire distance between the bar and the elbow] to represent the foot[-long section, while one] foot is divided to become an inch... The total length of the foot and inch [section] extends over one inch and 9 *fen*. Hence, one speaks of a foot and inch [section].[1]

In that classic, each of these three positions is believed to correspond to one of the twelve regular channels (*shi er zheng jing*). Since there are two hands, this immediately allows for 6 different possible positions. Then, if one divides each of these six positions into deep and shallow positions in terms of depth, one gets a total of 12 possible positions using the pulses on both wrists. The following representation shows the correspondences described in chapter 18 of the *Nan Jing* for these 12 pulse positions.

[1] *Nan Ching, op. cit.*, p. 81

		Right	Left
Cun	Superficial	Hand *yang ming*	Hand *tai yang*
	Deep	Hand *tai yin*	Hand *shao yin*
Guan	Superficial	Foot *yang ming*	Foot *shao yang*
	Deep	Foot *tai yin*	Foot *jue yin*
Chi	Superficial	Hand *shao yang*	Foot *tai yang*
	Deep	Hand *jue yin*	Foot *shao yin*

It is important to note that the *Nan Jing* uses hand and foot, yin and yang, six channel terminology when describing the correspondences of each of these 12 positions. This is significant because the *Nan Jing* is primarily an acupuncture text.

In chapter 18 of the *Nan Jing* the pulse at the *cun kou* is also divided into nine divisions from superficial to deep. The uppermost or most superficial section corresponds to heaven, the medium depth corresponds to humanity, and the deepest section corresponds to earth. However, the author of the *Nan Jing* states that in terms of disease, the heavenly section corresponds to diseases in the area from the chest upward to the head, the human section corresponds to diseases located between the diaphragm to the navel, and the earthly section corresponds to diseases located from below the navel to the feet. Since each of these three large sections can be divided into three sections, there are altogether 9 sections. When speaking of these, one can identify them by specifying the heaven of heaven section, the human of heaven section, the earth of heaven section, the heaven of human section, the human of human section, etc.

The above system is no longer used in modern TCM. It is still used by certain Japanese, Vietnamese, and Taiwanese acupuncturists as well as adherents of so-called Leamington Acupuncture developed by J. R. Worsley. It is presented here for reference and comparison purposes only.

In the first monograph on the pulse, written by Wang Shu-he (210-285 CE) and titled the *Mai Jing (Pulse Classic)*, the following correspondences are given. What is interesting to note here is that Wang ascribes the viscera and bowels connected to the hand and foot, yin and yang, six channels to the sections of the pulse the *Nan Jing* read as hand *tai yang*, etc. It is this representation of the correspondences between the viscera and bowels which formed the basis for most subsequent Chinese systems of pulse reading.

		Right	Left
Cun	Superficial	Large Intestine	Small Intestine
	Deep	Lungs	Heart
Guan	Superficial	Stomach	Gallbladder
	Deep	Spleen	Liver
Chi	Superficial	Triple Burner	Bladder
	Deep	Pericardium	Kidneys

Contemporary TCM pulse examination uses a slight variation of the above set of correspondences. This modern rendition is based on the *Bin Hu Mai Xue (The Lakeside Master's Study of the Pulse)*. This book is a compilation. The first section is based on the *Si Yan Ju Yao (Gathered Essentials in Four Characters)* written by Cui Jia-yan (420-479 CE). This was then re-edited by Li Yan-wen, the father of Li Shi-zhen. The second section, describing 27 pulse images and their definitions and indications in verse seems to have been added by Li Shi-zhen in 1564 CE. Because of the succinctness of these verses and their ease of memorization, this book has been used as a basic source for learning TCM pulse examination right up to this day.

One of the key differences between the system of correspondences in the *Bin Hu Mai Xue* and that of the *Nan Jing* and *Mai Jing* is that now the inch, bar, and cubit positions represent the upper, middle, and lower burners respectively. Thus each position may correspond to the main viscera or bowels in each of those three burners or any other body part located in each of those three burners. The anatomical locations of these three burners cover the same areas corresponding to the heaven, human, and earth sections of the pulse in the *Nan Jing*. In other words, the *cun* or inch position corresponds to everything from the bottom of the chest to the top of the head, the *guan* or bar position corresponds to the area of the body located between the diaphragm and the navel, and the *chi* or cubit position corresponds to everything below the navel.

In this system, no particular distinction is made in terms of correspondences depending upon depth. In other words, in the *guan* or bar position, it is not that the spleen is located deeper than the stomach. Whether one is feeling the spleen or the stomach depends on the pulse image in that position corroborated by the other signs and symptoms as well as the tongue and its coating. The representation below of pulse positions and their correspondences is taken from Zhang Jie-bin's *Jing Yue Quan Shu (Jing-yue's Complete Writings)* and is ultimately based on the *Bin Hu Mai Xue*. It represents the correspondences I use in my clinical practice.

	Right	Left
Cun	Lungs & center of chest (*Xiong Zhong*)	Heart & center of chest (*Dan Zhong*)
Guan	Spleen/stomach	Liver/gallbladder
Chi	Kidney & abdomen (L.I.)	Kidney & abdomen (Bladder & S.I.)

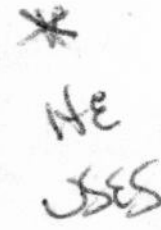

In the above rendition, it is interesting to note that the pulses on the right correspond to viscera and bowels which tend to have to do with yang qi and its engenderment and transformation, while the pulses on the left correspond to viscera and bowels which tend to have more to do with the engenderment and storage of yin blood and the transformation of fluids and humors. This is notwithstanding the fact that the *Bin Hu Mai Xue* points out that the left side is yang and the right side is yin.

The *Bin Hu Mai Xue* does also divide the depth of the pulse in general into three sections. The most superficial division corresponds to the heart and lungs, the middle division to the spleen and stomach, and the deepest section to the liver and kidneys. Other sources describe five divisions in terms of depth corresponding to the lungs, heart, spleen, liver, and kidneys going from superficial to deep respectively. However, I have never seen this system discussed in terms of clinical usage in any contemporary TCM source. Since the *Bin Hu Mai Xue* only mentions this system of correspondence but makes no further use of it, it is likely that its mention in that book is only a historical artifact and that it was not used in clinical practice even in the 16th century.

3
Feeling the Pulse Images

The Chinese medical literature has identified and named a number of pulse images (*mai xiang*) or types of pulse since at least the time of the *Nei Jing (Inner Classic*, circa 200 BCE). In that classic, 20 different pulse images are discussed. Zhang Zhong-jing (150?-219? CE), in his *Shang Han Lun (Treatise on Damage Due to Cold)/Jin Gui Yao Lue (Essentials of the Golden Cabinet)*, lists 22 pulse images. Wang Shu-he in his *Mai Jing (Pulse Classic)*, published sometime around 280 CE, lists 24 pulse images. Li Shi-zhen in the *Bin Hu Mai Xue (The Lakeside Master's Study of the Pulse)*, published in 1564 CE, describes 27 pulse images, while Li Zhong-zi, in his *Yi Zhong Bi Du (Essential Readings in Medicine)*, published in 1637 CE, discusses 28 pulse images. Today, most TCM texts discuss 27, 28, or 29 pulse images.

As stated in the Introduction, before one can feel any of these discreet pulse images, one must memorize their definitions. As Manfred Porkert points out, these definitions have been honed and refined over not less than 2000 years by 100 generations of educated, literate practitioners. Please do not simply read the following descriptions. It is absolutely essential that you memorize each and every one of them, word for word.

Normal & Disease Pulse Images

All pulse images can be divided into normal pulse images, called *ping mai*, literally a level pulse, and diseased pulse images, called *bing mai*. Before one can understand and feel diseased pulses, one must first know what are the characteristics of a normal, healthy pulse.

Ping Mai, the Normal Pulse

A *ping mai* has three characteristics:

1. *You shen*: It has spirit.

Its coming and going are distinct. It also has force. A pulse whose coming and going are indistinct and is minute, choppy, weak, or occasionally ceases is categorized as *wu shen*, without spirit.

2. *You wei*: It has stomach (qi).

This pulse is supple or flexible, harmonious, slippery, uninhibited, and not deep. If the pulse comes wiry, urgent, replete, or large or loses its suppleness and harmony, it is characterized as *wu wei qi*, without stomach qi. In ancient times, this was called the *zhen zang mai*, true visceral pulse, and was a sign of death.

3. *You gen*: It has root.

This refers to a pulse whose *chi*, cubit, or foot position can be felt all the way down to the bone. It is not floating. If a foot position pulse cannot be felt all the way down to the bone, it is called *wu gen*, without root.

If the *cun, guan,* and *chi* are neither floating nor deep but are harmonious and moderate, beat between 64-90 BPM, and have force (*you li*), this is a *ping mai*.

Bing Mai, Disease Pulses

Below are succinct definitions of 29 pulse images. At this stage in one's study, one should only concern oneself with the descriptions of each pulse. Later we will discuss the indications of each pulse and their combinations. These definitions are taken from the Chinese literature. Below each Chinese description, I have added my own comments, hopefully making these definitions all the more understandable.

1. ***Fu Mai*, Floating Pulse:** Located in the exterior. With finger raised, it has a surplus; when pressing down, it is insufficient. When pressure is released, it regains its full strength.

The floating pulse is sometimes also referred to in the English literature as the superficial pulse. The key to its discrimination is that it can be felt with light pressure, but, as pressure is increased, it disappears. When this pressure is let up, once again the pulse can be felt. Again if one presses down, the pulse does not persist to the root but disappears. Yet always, as pressure is released, the pulse reappears once again near the surface. The Chinese literature often likens this pulse to a piece of wood floating on water. However, that image is not as immediately clear and apprehendable as the fact that this pulse can be felt with light pressure but disappears with heavy pressure.

2. ***Chen Mai*, Deep Pulse:** Located near the bone. Cannot be detected with light or moderate pressure but can be felt with heavy pressure.

The deep pulse is just the opposite of the floating pulse. It cannot be felt near the surface with light pressure. One can only feel it as more pressure is exerted and the fingertips sink further down into the tissue. If one cannot feel the pulse with light pressure but can feel it with deeper pressure, then this is a deep pulse.

3. ***Chi Mai*, Slow Pulse:** Below 60 BPM or less than 4 beats per breath.

Traditionally, the rate of the pulse was gauged by the number of beats per cycle of respiration. However, the question then arises, whose respiration, the practitioner's or the patient's? Nowadays, it is easier to count the beats of the pulse while watching the second hand of one's wristwatch. Count for 15 seconds and then multiply by 4. This will give you the beats per minute or BPM. After one has felt pulses for awhile, one will immediately know if the pulse is fast or slow without having to look at one's watch.

4. ***Shu Mai*, Rapid Pulse:** Above 90 BPM or more than 5 beats per breath.

The fast pulse is self-explanatory. It refers to a pulse which beats more than 90 beats per minute. Like the slow pulse, after a short while, one will immediately know if a pulse is fast or not.

5. ***Xu Mai,* Vacuous Pulse:** A) A generalized term for various types of forceless pulses. B) A slow, large floating, empty, vacuous, soft, forceless pulse image.

Some Chinese authors and practitioners only use the term vacuous pulse as a generalized name for all types of forceless pulse. However, others do see the vacuous pulse as a discreet pulse image. In that case, its key features are that it is slow, floating, large, and forceless.

6. ***Shi Mai,* Replete Pulse:** A) A generalized term for various types of forceful pulses. B) A long-bodied, wiry, large, hard, and replete pulse which has a surplus either floating or deep.

Like the vacuous pulse, some regard the replete pulse as only a generalized term for a variety of forceful pulses. When it is seen as a discreet pulse image, its key points are that it is long, large, wiry, and forceful.

7. ***Kou Mai,* Scallion-stalk Pulse:** Floating, soft, large body, but empty center; feels like a scallion leaf.

This pulse is traditionally likened to a scallion leaf. A scallion leaf is hollow in its center. This pulse can be felt superficially. However, it is soft, *i.e.*, not forceful, and large. Further, when pressure is applied, it disappears rapidly and completely.

8. ***Xian Mai,* Wiry Pulse:** Fine, long, has strength, feels like a lute wire.

The wiry pulse is traditionally compared to the feeling of one's fingers on a lute string. It is fine, long, and forceful. Sometimes this wiry quality only reveals itself when one changes pressure or rolls one's fingers slightly up and down the pulse. In other words, it is not an always immediately perceptible quality when present but sometimes must be searched for. This is one of the few pulses which must be pointed out to the student by an experienced practitioner. However, it is an extremely common pulse image and, therefore, there are no lack of models with this pulse. Once it is pointed out and felt for oneself, it is like sugar in one's mouth. From that time forward one immediately knows what a wiry pulse is like.

9. ***Hong Mai*, Surging Pulse:** Floating, large; comes on exuberant, departs debilitated.

The surging pulse is one of the floating pulses. Therefore, first of all it is rootless. Secondly it is large. Traditionally it is likened to a wave coming onto the shore with force but retreating without force. That description has never meant much to me. Therefore I recommend concentrating on the fact that the surging pulse is a large, floating pulse.

10. ***Wei Mai*, Faint Pulse:** Insufficient, extremely fine, soft, barely palpable. It may sometimes be felt and then sometimes it is lost.

The key to feeling a faint pulse is that it is very, very fine and forceless. It is barely palpable and even when one has found it, it may sometimes be lost again.

11. ***Chang Mai*, Long Pulse:** Long, can be felt beyond its own location or range.

The long pulse refers to a pulse which can be felt further up the forearm than usual. If one slides their ring finger resting on the *chi* or cubit section up the forearm, one can feel that the pulse persists distinctly further than is usual in most people.

12. ***Duan Mai*, Short Pulse:** Does not reach (*i.e.*, fill longitudinally) its location or range.

The short pulse is just the opposite of the long pulse. While the long pulse continues proximally up the arm from the *chi* or cubit section, the short pulse only reaches distally to the *guan* or bar position. In other words, it does not reach the *cun* or inch section.

13. *Hua Mai,* Slippery Pulse: Comes smoothly flowing and uninhibited; feels smooth like pearls rolling in a dish.

The traditional description of a pearl rolling in a dish has always been a hard one for me to grasp. The slippery pulse is another one of the very pulses which must be pointed out by an experienced practitioner. Once one feels a slippery pulse, then its slippery quality is quite self-evident. Literally one can feel its slipperiness, its rolling quality.

14. *Se Mai,* Choppy Pulse: Slow, relaxed, stagnant, difficult, fine, small, short, may stop and lose a beat but then recovers. It is not smoothly flowing. It feels like a piece of bamboo scraped by a knife.

The choppy pulse is one about which there is great confusion. Again, its traditional likening of a knife scraping across a piece of bamboo is not very revealing. First of all, in feeling the choppy pulse, one must understand that it is a relaxed or slow and fine pulse. Secondly, although it is not classified as an interrupted pulse, there is variability to its rate and rhythm. The pulse seems to slow down and then speed up, and not every beat hits one's fingertips with the same force. Literally, the word *se* means astringent, but choppy is a much better functional translation. Some practitioners call this a 3/5 pulse because sometimes it comes with 3 beats per respiration and sometimes 5. In any case, one should look for slowing down and then speeding up. This is what the Chinese are referring to when they describe this pulse's movement as stagnant, difficult, and not smoothly flowing.

15. *Jin Mai,* Tight Pulse: Tight, has strength, feels like a taut rope.

Many practitioners have trouble distinguishing a tight pulse from a wiry pulse. Both have tensile strength or force. However, the wiry pulse is a fine pulse and the tight pulse is not fine. Therefore, the size and strength of the tight pulse are greater than the wiry pulse.

16. *Huan Mai,* Moderate or Relaxed Pulse: A) As a *ping mai*, level or normal pulse; it is harmonious, relaxed, and forceful. B) As a *bing mai* or diseased pulse, it is relaxed, loose, slack, and on the verge of slow. It comes right at about 60 BPM.

The moderate pulse can either refer to a normal, healthy pulse which is not wiry or tight, or it may refer to a disease pulse. As a disease pulse, this pulse is not uncommonly felt in clinical practice. It is not slow but it is on the verge of being slow.

17. *Fu Mai,* Hidden Pulse: Difficult to feel, under the sinews, not obvious, requires heavy pressure to the bone to obtain.

This is a difficult to find pulse. It is even deeper than the deep pulse. However, it is different from the faint pulse in that the faint pulse is difficult to find because it is so small, weak, and evanescent. In other words, the faint pulse is not necessarily deep. The hidden pulse must be found very deep and close to the bone. In addition, this pulse is not large or strong.

18. *Xi Mai,* Fine Pulse: Soft, feels like a silken thread, weak, without strength, but persistent.

The fine pulse, also referred to in the English literature as the thready pulse, is extremely common, especially in female patients. It feels like a thread. It is not very forceful, but it is continuous and is not scattered by pressure.

19. *Jie Mai,* Bound Pulse: Slow, relaxed, stops at irregular intervals.

The bound pulse is one of several interrupted pulses. The key to distinguishing it from those other interrupted pulses is that it is relaxed or slow and it stops at irregular intervals. If one feels that the pulse is skipping beats, one must first decide if the pulse is fast or slow, relaxed or normal in rate. Secondly, one should count the beats. If the pulse is relaxed or slow and the pause between beats comes at irregular intervals, then this is the bound pulse.

20. *Ruo Mai,* Weak Pulse: Deep, fine, soft like thread.

The weak pulse is made up of three qualities. It is deep, not superficial. It is fine, not large. And it is relatively forceless.

21. *Ruan Mai,* Soft Pulse (*Ru Mai,* Soggy Pulse): Floating, fine, soft, and flexible. Can be felt with light pressure but cannot be obtained by heavy pressure.

This pulse may be called by either of two names, the soggy pulse or the soft pulse. This is another of the commonly encountered pulses in Western clinical practice and it is extremely important that one be able to identify it. First of all, this is a floating pulse. Secondly, it is fine. And third, it is relatively forceless. Once one memorizes those three qualities or characteristics, one can feel this pulse.

22. *Dai Mai,* Regularly Interrupted Pulse: Comparatively relaxed and weak; stops at regular intermittent intervals. These intervals may be strikingly long.

Like the bound pulse, the regularly interrupted pulse is relaxed in rate. However, whereas the bound pulse skips beats at irregular intervals, the regularly interrupted pulse skips beats at regular intervals. This means that if one counts the beats, the pause comes after every so many beats; for instance, 1, 2, 3, 4, pause, 1, 2, 3, 4, pause, 1, 2, 3, 4, pause, etc. In addition, these pauses can be surprisingly and even frighteningly long.

23. *Ge Mai,* Drumskin Pulse: Wiry and large with an empty center; feels like the head of a drum.

The drumskin pulse is also a floating pulse. Like the scallion-stalk pulse, it is both large and empty in its center. That means that when one pushes down with more pressure, the pulse disappears. However, unlike the scallion-stalk pulse, it is a wiry, floating pulse. If one remembers that the drumskin pulse is 1) floating, 2) large, and 3) wiry, then one can feel it in clinical practice.

24. ***Lao Mai,*** **Confined Pulse:** Pressed superficially or moderately, does not respond, but can be obtained by heavy pressure. Hard, firm, not changeable, replete, large, wiry, and long.

The confined pulse is a deep pulse. However, unlike the hidden pulse, in that deep position, it is large, wiry, forceful, and long.

25. ***San Mai,*** **Scattered Pulse:** It is floating, large, and without root; with light pressure, it is easily changeable, becoming scattered and chaotic. Heavy pressure leads to its absence.

The scattered pulse is yet another of the floating pulses. Like the hollow and drumskin pulses, it is also large. However, its distinguishing characteristic is that even with light pressure its beat becomes changeable. If heavier pressure is applied, it disappears altogether.

26. ***Dong Mai,*** **Stirring Pulse:** Slippery, rapid, forceful; feels like a (jumping) bean.

The stirring pulse is a form of slippery pulse. However, it is slippery, rapid, and forceful. As long as one keeps these three characteristics in mind, they will be able to feel the stirring pulse.

27. ***Cu Mai,*** **Skipping or Rapid Irregularly Interrupted Pulse:** Rapidand irregularly interrupted.

The skipping pulse is another of the interrupted pulses. Its distinguishing qualities are that it is rapid, not relaxed or slow, and that it skips at irregular intervals. Therefore, of the three interrupted pulses, the bound, regularly interrupted, and the skipping pulses, the skipping pulse is the only one which is rapid.

28. ***Da Mai,*** **Large Pulse:** Large, fills up fingertip, forceful.

The large pulse is exactly like its name implies. It is large. However, this largeness does not refer to its longitudinal quality but to its breadth.

Another way to describe this pulse is that it is wide. In addition, it is forceful.

29. ***Ji Mai*****, Racing Pulse:** Very rapid, over 120 BPM or 7-8 BPM.

The racing pulse is not all that commonly seen in Western clinical practice which tends to be entirely out-patient oriented. However, it is a very easy pulse to remember and distinguish. It is a rapid pulse. But it is not just an ordinary rapid pulse. It is a *very* rapid pulse. The racing pulse beats more than 120 beats per minute.

The Four Basic Pulse Images

The *Bin Hu Mai Xue (Lakeside Master's Study of the Pulse)* states that there are four principal or essential pulse images. These are:

1. Floating
2. Deep
3. Slow
4. Rapid

Zhu Dan-xi reiterates this fact in the *Ge Zhi Yu Lun (Extra Treatises Based on Investigation & Inquiry)* when he says:

> The diseases in human beings fall into four [categories], known as cold, heat, repletion, and vacuity. Therefore, the student of the pulse should take the floating, deep, slow, and rapid [pulses] as the reins in observing disease conditions. This is an unchanging principle.[1]

Whether a pulse is slow or rapid in beat is extremely easy to determine. Likewise, after one understands what floating and deep mean in terms of Chinese pulse examination, these are also very easy to check for. Most of the above 29 pulse images are combinations of one or more of these basic four qualities with one or more other qualities. Thus most of these 29 pulse images can be categorized as types of either floating or deep, slow or rapid

[1] Zhu Dan-xi, *Extra Treatises Based on Investigation & Inquiry*, trans. by Yang Shou-zhong & Duan Wu-jin, Blue Poppy Press, Boulder, CO, 1994, p. 13

pulses. The chart below shows how most of the above pulses can be categorized.

Floating	Deep	Slow	Rapid
Floating	Deep	Slow	Rapid
Hollow or scallion-stalk	Hidden	Bound	Skipping
Drumskin	Confined	Regularly intermittent	Racing
Soft or soggy	Weak	Choppy	Stirring
Vacuous			
Surging			
Scattered			

The four qualities of slow or rapid, floating or deep are extremely easy to differentiate. By knowing whether a pulse is slow or fast, floating or deep, one can immediately narrow down the list of possible pulse images when examining an individual patient's pulse. If a pulse is floating, then it can only be a floating pulse, scallion-stalk pulse, drumskin pulse, soggy pulse, vacuous pulse, surging pulse, or scattered pulse. If the pulse is deep, then it can only be a deep pulse, hidden pulse, confined pulse, or weak pulse. If the pulse is slow, it can only be a slow pulse, bound pulse, regularly intermittent pulse, or a choppy pulse. However, all of the last three are irregular in beat, either skipping beats or speeding up and slowing down. If the pulse is rapid, it can only be a rapid pulse, skipping pulse, racing pulse, or stirring pulse. To distinguish a rapid pulse from a racing pulse, all one has to do is count the beats, while a skipping pulse does just that, skips beats. A stirring pulse is not only rapid but slippery and forceful.

Distinguishing between such basic pairs of opposites is called *dui dai* in Chinese or contrasting. Besides the dichotomies of floating and deep and fast and slow, one may also contrast the slippery pulse to the choppy pulse. One comes uninhibitedly and the other comes stagnantly and with difficulty as if overcoming some obstacle. Likewise one can contrast the long and short pulse and those pulses which have force (*you li*) with those that are relatively forceless (*wu li*). The forceful pulses are the replete, wiry, tight, stirring, slippery, confined, long, and large pulses. The forceless pulses are the minute, fine, weak, vacuous, hollow, scattered, soggy, and regularly interrupted pulses.

When feeling the pulse, one should ask oneself a series of questions in a very methodical, step by step manner:

1. Is the pulse fast or slow?
2. Is the pulse floating or deep?
3. Does the pulse have force or not?
4. Is the pulse long or short?

These are very simple questions. The answers to them are all easy and immediate. One can tell if a pulse is fast or slow by counting the beats. One can tell if a pulse is floating or deep by its response to pressure. One can tell if a pulse is forceful or forceless also by its response to pressure. And one can tell if a pulse is long by whether it can be felt proximal to the cubit or *chi* position and if it is short by whether it reaches the inch or *cun* position.

If the pulse is floating, then one must see what other qualities it has. Is it fine and floating? If so, is it fine, floating, and comparatively weak or soft? If it is, then that is the soft or soggy pulse. Is it deep? If so, is it deep, wiry, and forceful? If so, it is the hidden pulse.

This is actually quite a simple and straightforward process. However, one cannot even begin this process with only a vague idea of the definitions of these pulse images. If one feels the pulse and does not know what adjective to use, then, in the overwhelming majority of cases seen in the out-patient clinic, there are only either of two problems: either 1) they have not learned these pulse images' descriptions or 2) they are not actively analyzing the pulse characteristics in terms of these images.

In addition, there are two other adjectives that are important when attempting to use the above 29 pulse images in clinical practice. These two adjectives are *wei*, slightly, and *shen*, very. One person's pulse may be only slightly wiry, while another person's may be very wiry. Someone's pulse may be very fine. Another person's may be very slippery.

Terminology & the Pulse Images

As quoted above, one of the reasons that Manfred Porkert is insistent on memorizing the descriptions of the 27-29 pulse images is so one can "communicate to his colleagues what he feels." Another, related current impediment to Western practitioners mastering Chinese pulse examination is the confusion of translational terminology used to describe pulse images. In Chinese, every TCM practitioner from Urumuqi to Fuzhou, from Xizang to Harbin, and from Beijing to Guangzhou uses the same words for these 27-29 standard pulse images. A *hua mai* is a *hua mai* in Shanghai, Nanjing, and Shijiazhuang. In the English language literature, however, some people call the *hua mai* a slippery pulse, a rolling pulse, a gliding pulse, or a smooth pulse. Therefore, when students and even practitioners go from reading one book or another or from studying with one teacher or another, they have no way of knowing whether the smooth pulse in one place is the same as the slippery pulse in another. This makes it, therefore, very hard to cross-reference information and the result is confusion.

Therefore, throughout this book I have used Nigel Wiseman's translational terminology. I do this not because I like it or agree with every one of his choices. I certainly like barrier better than bar for *guan* and foot better than cubit for *chi*. I also like flooding better than surging for *hong mai*. However, if one uses such a standard translational terminology and if anyone is confused or curious as to what the actual Chinese character is, they can easily look it up in Wiseman's *Glossary*. Therefore, I highly recommend that when students and teachers speak about pulse images and when practitioners write down pulse images in their charts, they either use the Pinyin romanization of the Chinese or they use a terminology that can easily be referenced to the Chinese characters.

In other words, there is already enough confusion about Chinese pulse examination without everyone being additionally confused about whether one is talking about this pulse or that. If one gets used to using the Pinyin, perhaps that is the best and safest way. For those who are resistant to that, then please consider Wiseman's terminology. Even though many of Weisman's terms may sound peculiar, at least they are unambiguous, because one can easily reference their characters

4
The Technique of Examining the Pulse

In TCM, there is what is referred to as the physical technique of examining the pulse. In Chinese, this is referred to as *cao zong*, manipulation. Most modern Chinese and English books on TCM diagnosis discuss this method before describing the pulse images. However, I strongly agree with Manfred Porkert that before one learns to physically feel the pulse one must memorize the basic definitions of the main pulse images. However, once one has memorized the basic pulse images, then one does need to know something about the actual physical technique of examining the pulse.

Time

The *Su Wen (Simple Questions)* states, "The pulse should be taken in the early morning."[1] This is because in the early morning one has not yet been subjected to all of the influences that go to make up one's daily life. In addition, it is traditionally believed that yin and yang are relatively in balance macrocosmically just before dawn. In fact, when the *Su Wen* says the pulse should be examined in the early morning, this meant that time just before sunrise when the eastern sky is filled with light but the sun has not yet crossed the horizon. This means that the patient has only recently risen and they have not yet eaten, engaged in work or other physical activity, had sex, etc.

---

1 Quoted in *Fundamentals of Chinese Medicine*, trans. by Nigel Wiseman and Andy Ellis, Paradigm Publications, Brookline, MA, 1985, p. 142

Although these are the traditional teachings, they are more than a little difficult to follow in modern Western clinical practice. In point of fact, one can take the pulse at any time of the day. However, when one does take the pulse, they should take into account that the pulse is affected by the diurnal cycle and such things as eating, emotional upsetment, physical activity, etc. One should, therefore, question the patient briefly about their recent activities—how long ago they ate, did they have to hurry to the office, did someone upset them emotionally before coming for their appointment, did they drive in traffic—and, if there is some recent strong influence that might skew or alter the pulse image, one simply takes that into account in their examination.

Posture

The patient can be either seated upright or lying down on their back. The forearm should be horizontal and held slightly below the level of the heart. The palm of the hand should be face up and the wrist should be held straight and kept relaxed. This is best achieved by providing a small cushion or pad on which the patient may rest their wrist. If the patient holds their arm in a stiff or unnatural position or if the arm is held up above the level of the heart, one may not get a true reading of the pulse.

Breathing

As was pointed out in the Introduction, it is believed that respiration is associated with the movement of the pulse. Therefore, it is important that the patient's breathing be relaxed and normal. However, because in antiquity, the practitioner's respiration was the standard for measuring beats per breathing respiration, it is also considered traditionally important for the practitioner's breathing to be relaxed and unconstrained.

Finger Placement & Movement

When examining the pulse in TCM, the practitioner should feel the *cun* or inch position with their index finger, the *guan* or bar position with their middle finger, and the *chi* or cubit position with their ring finger. One should first press gently and then press harder or alternate gentle and heavy pressure repeatedly so as to differentiate the qualities of the pulse. *Ju, an, tui*, and *xun* are four verbs in Chinese which are used to describe the methods of varying pressure and moving one's fingertips during pulse examination. *Ju an* means to apply and release pressure. Releasing or lifting, one is able to feel the pulse at its most superficial. Pressing, one can feel the pulse deeper down. *Tui xun* means to push and search. This refers to moving the fingers sideways up and down the pulse longitudinally. This tells about length and is also important in determining a slightly wiry pulse.

There are also two techniques of examining the pulse depending on whether one feels all three positions at one time or whether one feels each position separately. *Zong an* or simultaneous palpation refers to feeling all three positions with all three fingers at the same time. *Dan an*, individual palpation means feeling only one position with a single finger at a time. Usually, one uses both techniques when examining the pulse. Simultaneous palpation tells the practitioner the dominant or overall images of the pulse, while individual palpation is used to clarify the precise pulse images present at particular positions.

Duration of Examination

Wiseman translates *chu chi* as initial palpation. However, it may also be translated as transitory palpation. This refers to examining the pulse for only a short period of time, usually less than a minute. Such transitory palpation is often sufficient in clinical practice. If the patient comes in for the treatment of a common cold with a sore throat, fever, no sweating, slight chills, stuffed nose, and a slight cough, one merely needs to feel the pulse to confirm that this is indeed a wind heat superficial invasion. Unless there are other signs and symptoms that make the practitioner think that something much more complicated is going on with this patient, to belabor the pulse, extracting every possible nuance would be a waste of time and energy, about which I will have more to say.

Jiu chi means extended palpation. It refers to a relatively long period of examining the pulse, from several to 15 minutes or more. Such prolonged examination is important in establishing a patient's constitutional pulse or for parsing out complicated patterns.

Cultivating Stillness During Pulse Examination

In Chinese, *zhi mu* can be translated as the eyes of the fingers or finger-eyes. It means the most sensitive part of the pads of the fingertips. However, it also implies that the practitioner must develop eyes in their fingertips. Basically, in order to examine the pulse accurately, one must achieve a calm but alert state of mind. One must be able to put their mind in their fingertips so that they can feel the physical sensations that pressing the radial arteries provokes. In addition, they must also be able to intelligently and methodically search for and discriminate among these physical sensations without either becoming so calm as to fall asleep or so alert as to become distracted by other sounds, sights, and thoughts.

It is my experience that pulse examination is a form of meditation, and the practice of meditation can greatly help in developing one's abilities to examine the pulse. This does not imply that one's reading of the pulse is based on mystical insight. It only means that one must be able to calm one's thoughts, fears, hopes, desires, and preconceptions in order to concentrate on fairly subtle physical sensations at the same time as being able to logically think about those physical feelings. I personally find it helpful to close my eyes to achieve the kind of concentration necessary for putting my eyes in my fingers.

The type of stillness I am talking about is definitely an active stillness and does require an expenditure of energy. Therefore, one should not be surprised or alarmed that they cannot focus their mind and gather up that kind of energy all day, every day, day after day for every patient who comes to the clinic. As mentioned above, some cases require relatively transitory palpation and others require more prolonged palpation and examination. Nonetheless, one should be warned not to attempt to diagnose more patients per day than their mental and physical energies will allow. Here in the United States of America it is the legal responsibility of the practitioner to only schedule as many patients to whom they can give professionally competent care. This legal requirement could have interesting ramifications when it comes to Chinese pulse examination.

5
Interpreting the Pulse

Having decided what qualities or images the pulse actually presents, the next step is the interpretation of those images. This means deciding what those images mean diagnostically, what they indicate. Although these images tend to appear in combinations, one should first understand the underlying mechanisms and then their diagnostic indications separately before looking at more complex pulse image combinations.

One of the things that I have noticed in students and young practitioners when it comes to pulse examination is that they tend to remember only the first of typically several possible indications. Thus when presented with a floating pulse, they immediately jump to the conclusion that the patient is suffering from an exterior condition. Although they may be exhibiting an exterior condition, there are other reasons why the pulse may be floating. As I have already commented, here in the West, we typically see chronic, complicated cases. Therefore, commonly, it is the second or third indication of a pulse image, not its first and most frequently mentioned or repeated indication that actually is important in our patients' pulses.

One of the best ways that I have found to remember and understand the indications of the various pulse images is to understand the underlying mechanisms responsible for their production. A pulse may have two or three indications, yet still there is usually some commonality in their disease mechanisms as they affect the pulse that explains why these diverse patterns or disease mechanisms produce the same pulse image.

The Underlying Mechanisms of the Pulse Images

1. ***Fu Mai*, Floating Pulse:** The floating pulse can be felt superficially but not on deep pressure. Here the pulse represents the qi. Therefore, a floating or superficial pulse means that the qi is either high up in the body or gathered in the exterior. Therefore, there are several mechanisms for the production of a floating pulse. First, an external evil may have invaded the body and is currently lodged in the exterior defensive or *wai wei*. In this case, the body's righteous qi struggles with the evil qi in the exterior. In addition, such externally invading qi typically attacks the upper part of the body first.

Secondly, if there is insufficient yin, yang qi may counterflow upward and outward. This is due to the inherent nature of yang qi. Thus the pulse is felt to be floating since this corresponds to the exterior and upper parts of the body.

Third, it is also possible for qi or yang vacuity to lose its root in the lower origin. In that case, yang qi may also float upward and to the surface, thus producing a floating pulse.

Deciding which of these mechanisms is responsible for a given floating pulse depends upon the other corroborating signs and symptoms. For instance, if there are fever, stuffed nose, slight cough, and a sore throat all of recent onset and the pulse is floating and rapid with a thin, white tongue coating or slight yellow tongue coating, these other signs and symptoms confirm that this floating pulse is due to an external invasion lodged in the exterior, whereas, if there is a red tongue tip, a scanty or thin, yellow tongue coating, tidal fever, heat in the five hearts, night sweats, dizziness, tinnitus, and a floating, fine, and rapid pulse, then this all adds up to vacuity heat counterflowing upward and outward due to yin vacuity. And if there are cold feet, clear, long urination, low back and knee soreness and weakness, low-grade fever, a light red tongue or a red tongue tip, flushed cheeks, and a floating, slow, large, and forceless pulse, this is upward and outwardly counterflowing yang qi which has lost its root in its lower origin.

2. *Chen Mai,* Deep Pulse: As stated above, the depth of the pulse tells the practitioner something about the patient's yang qi. If there is a deep pulse, it means that the patient's yang qi is in the interior and/or lower parts of their body. This may be due to several reasons. Either there is not enough yang qi to push the pulse upward or something is obstructing the free flow of the yang qi so that it cannot move upward and outward. Thus a deep pulse may be due to yang qi vacuity or evil qi lodged in the interior or lower parts of the body. In the second case, the body's yang qi is concentrated internally or below where it struggles with the evil qi.

3. *Chi Mai,* Slow Pulse: The rate of the stirring or beating of the pulse is also a function of yang qi. Thus the rate of beating of the pulse tells the practitioner primarily about the presence or absence of heat in the body. Thus a slow pulse is usually an indication of cold. This cold can be either replete or vacuity and located in the exterior or interior. The exact nature of the cold and its cause and location are determined by the other qualities of the pulse. For instance, a slow, tight, forceful pulse indicates replete cold, while a slow, fine, forceless pulse indicates vacuity cold.

The reader should also be aware that cold can also produce a tight pulse. In other words, there may be cold in the body without a slow pulse. For instance, there may be a floating, tight pulse in the inch or *cun* position. The floating pulse suggests that there is an exterior pattern, while the tight pulse indicates that there is exterior cold. In addition, the tight pulse also indicates that there is pain due to cold congelation in the upper body, such as headache and upper back and shoulder tightness and pain.

4. *Shu Mai,* Rapid Pulse: If the pulse is faster than normal, this means that there is more heat in the body than normal. This heat may be due to repletion or vacuity and that is determined by other simultaneous pulse images and other signs and symptoms. For instance, if there is phlegm heat, the phlegm may cause the pulse to be slippery and the heat may cause it to be rapid. (In actuality, as we will see below, the heat will also cause the pulse to be slippery.) In any case, if there is vacuity heat, the pulse will tend to be fine and rapid or floating and rapid.

5. *Xi Mai,* Fine Pulse: Fineness describes the volume of the contents of the pulse. The contents of the pulse or channels and vessels are the qi, blood, and body fluids. Therefore, the underlying disease mechanism of a fine pulse is qi and blood vacuity weakness. Although most textbooks use the words qi and blood, the reader should also know that this can include blood and yin.

6. *Hua Mai,* Slippery Pulse: It is said that the slippery pulse is produced by blood swirling through the channels and vessels. Therefore, the slippery pulse can simply be a normal pulse showing that there is abundant qi and blood and that this qi and blood is flowing uninhibitedly.

However, it can also be the manifestation of phlegm, dampness, and stagnant food or of heat. In terms of phlegm and dampness, both of these have a common source. That source is the ability of the spleen to transport and transform fluids and humors. If the spleen loses its command over transportation and transformation, these fluids gather and turn into dampness and eventually congeal into phlegm. However, this also means that there are more fluids and humors flowing in the channels and vessels than normal and hence the slippery pulse. In actual fact, because dampness is usually due to spleen vacuity and because the spleen is the latter heaven or postnatal root of qi and blood engenderment and transformation, frequently the pulse becomes fine and not slippery when there is gathering of dampness. It is mostly when there is phlegm dampness or damp heat that the pulse becomes slippery in response to dampness.

The spleen and stomach are also responsible for transforming food and liquids into the finest essence. In the case of food stagnation, the spleen and stomach are not capable of completing this transformation. Thus the qi and fluids of food and liquids enter the channels and vessels untransformed, increasing the contents of the vessels and also making the pulse slippery.

Heat is nothing but a lot of qi in a small area, and it is qi that is responsible for the movement and propulsion of the blood. Therefore, heat forces the blood to move. This increased movement can then produce the swirling blood pulse we call slippery.

7. *Xian Mai*, Wiry Pulse: The wiry pulse is a constricted, constrained pulse. It occurs when the qi is not able to spread properly. This is called the orderly reaching of the qi. This may be due to several reasons. First and foremost, due to emotional stress, anger, resentment, and frustration, the liver may lose its command over coursing and discharge. Thus the qi does not reach orderly, flow freely, or flow smoothly. Secondly, dampness may impede the flow of qi. Dampness is a yin evil and qi is yang. This yin may impede the free flow of yang qi. And third, blood vacuity may also result in a wiry pulse. The blood is the mother of the qi. If blood becomes vacuous, the qi loses its moisture and nourishment. Thus its free flow also becomes unsmooth. In clinical practice, it is a fact that liver depression, qi stagnation frequently, even typically, exists with simultaneous blood vacuity and spleen dampness. That is the rationale behind the composition of the most famous formula for treating liver depression, qi stagnation, *Xiao Yao San* (Rambling Powder).

8. *Duan Mai*, Short Pulse: The short pulse is defined as one which does not reach beyond the bar or *guan* position. As stated above, the three positions, inch, bar, and cubit, respectively correspond to the upper, middle, and lower burners. Thus if the qi cannot reach to the inch position, this means that the central or middle qi is insufficient. This is an easy pulse image to identify and also usually an easy pattern to remedy.

9. *Jin Mai*, Tight Pulse: A tight pulse is like a wiry pulse but is larger and more forceful. In part this is because the wiry pulse is usually associated with an element of blood vacuity. Like the wiry pulse, the tight pulse is an inhibited pulse showing lack of free flow. There are usually two mechanisms responsible for the manifestation of a tight pulse. First, if it is axiomatic that heat forces the blood to move, it is also axiomatic that cold causes the blood to congeal. Thus a tight pulse may be due to cold congelation inhibiting free flow. Secondly, when a person experiences severe pain, it is a natural reaction to tense or contract. Hence a tense pulse may also be caused as a reaction to severe pain.

10. *Huan Mai*, Relaxed Pulse: As a disease pulse, the relaxed pulse is on the verge of being slow. As we have said above, the speed of the pulse is a function of yang qi since it is qi which propels the blood and is responsible for the stirring or beating of the pulse. Thus a relaxed pulse is usually due to qi vacuity not pushing the blood as quickly as it should. Since it is the heart which controls the blood, meaning that it is the heart which propels the blood, a relaxed pulse is frequently a sign of heart qi vacuity. Since the heart and spleen qi are closely related, it may also be due to a heart/spleen dual vacuity.

11. ***Ru Mai*, Soggy Pulse:** The soggy pulse or soft pulse (*ruan mai*) is defined as a fine, floating, soft, *i.e.*, not very forceful, pulse. The soggy pulse may be due either to qi and blood vacuity or to a gathering of dampness. If due to qi and blood vacuity, it is fine and floating because of insufficient blood to root the qi and it is soft or forceless due to insufficient qi, the source of force. In fact, I believe that the soft, soggy pulse due to accumulation of dampness is due to this very same mechanism with the added proviso that, due to the spleen's loss of command over transportation and transformation, dampness and water spill over into the space between the skin and flesh.

12. ***Xu Mai*, Vacuous Pulse, *Hong Mai*, Surging Pulse, *Kou Mai*, Scallion-stalk Pulse, *Gu Mai*, Drumskin Pulse & *San Mai*, Scattered Pulse:** These are all varieties of floating pulses. Thus they are due to counterflow of yang qi upward and outward. Qi counterflows upward and outward either because it has lost its root in the blood, yin, or the kidneys or due to heat whose nature is to move upward and outward. The surging pulse is due not just to vacuity but also to the presence of heat. The drumskin pulse is not just due to qi vacuity but also to blood and essence vacuity and so it is also wiry. The drumskin pulse is associated with immanent qi desertion, and so it is weak and forceless.

13. ***Fu Mai*, Hidden Pulse & *Lao Mai*, Confined Pulse:** The hidden and confined pulses are both types of deep pulses. This means that yang qi is not able to rise upward as is its nature. The hidden pulse is deep because of qi stagnation and blood stasis blocking its free flow. The confined pulse is stronger than the hidden pulse. However, it is also wiry. Thus it too is an

inhibited pulse. Because it is strong, it is not due to vacuity but rather to cold damp congelation and stagnation.

14. *Wei Mai,* Faint Pulse & *Rou Mai,* Weak Pulse: The faint pulse is an extremely small, weak, and evanescent pulse. It tends to disappear with even slight pressure. Its mechanism is extreme qi and blood vacuity. The weak pulse is also fine and forceless but it is also deep. Its depth is due to insufficient qi to raise clear yang.

15. *Cu Mai,* Skipping Pulse: The skipping pulse has two main characteristics. First it is rapid. This rapidity is due to heat. Secondly it skips beats irregularly. This is because there is blockage and obstruction. This blockage may be due to qi, blood, phlegm, or food.

16. *Jie Mai,* Bound Pulse: The bound pulse is a relaxed or slow pulse which skips a beat at irregular intervals. It can be due to main mechanisms. First, if actually slow, it is due to cold. In that case, the skipping is due to cold congelation causing stasis which in turns impedes the free flow of qi and blood. Secondly, if it is just relaxed, this is usually due to heart qi vacuity complicated by or causing blood stasis. The relaxed quality is due to qi vacuity not propelling the qi and blood which then become stopped and static. This static blood then impedes the free flow of what qi and blood there is.

17. *Se Mai,* Choppy Pulse: The choppy pulse is also an inhibited pulse. The qi and blood do not flow freely and thus the pulse tends to be relaxed or slowish. Since they do not flow smoothly, they tend to speed up and slow down as if flowing against resistance and therefore by fits and starts. However, the choppy pulse may also be due to blood vacuity and fluid and humor insufficiency. If the blood and body fluids are insufficient to moisten and nourish the vessels, the qi and blood cannot flow freely through those channels and vessels. In actual fact, qi stagnation and blood stasis tend to damage the blood and body fluids since static blood prevents the engenderment and transformation of fresh blood, while qi and blood vacuity often evolve into blood stasis. Thus the choppy pulse is not so much due to either stasis and stagnation or vacuity weakness as a combination of both.

18. *Ji Mai,* Racing Pulse: The racing pulse is nothing other than an extremely fast rapid pulse. Its mechanisms are extreme heat and consumption of yin.

19. *Dong Mai,* Stirring Pulse: The stirring pulse is also a rapid pulse. However, it is rapid, slippery, forceful, and wiry. This means that it is moving more than is normal but is also being restrained at the same time. Ted Kaptchuk states that the rapidity of the stirring pulse is not due to heat. Textbooks describe the mechanisms at work as yin and yang fighting with each other. This fighting is between pain or anything else that causes constriction and wiriness in the pulse, and fright. The pain causes the tension or the contraction, *i.e.*, the wiriness, while the fright causes the qi to move chaotically. It comes apart from the yin blood and jumps ahead, pushing the pulse more rapidly.

20. *Shi Mai,* Replete Pulse: This is a large, wiry, forceful pulse. The mechanism of its production is the struggle between replete evil qi and relatively strong righteous qi. The pulse is wiry because this struggle is impeding the free and uninhibited flow of qi and blood.

Common Factors Affecting the Pulse

Once one understands, according to the theories and mechanisms of TCM how the main pulse images are created, one must also know what factors must be taken into account when interpreting the pulse. TCM is based on the same theory of ceaseless change which underlies the *Yi Jing (Classic of Change)*. Macrocosmically, everything is changing on the outside. There is the progression of the season, the cycle of the moon, the diurnal rhythm, and constant changes in weather. Microcosmically, everyone is different from everyone else. What is normal for one person is abnormal for another. Thus one must always factor into their interpretation of the pulse various modifying influences. The main factors influencing the pulse which need to be taken into consideration are: age, sex, body type, lifestyle, anatomical variation, and seasonal variation.

Age

The younger the age, the faster the pulse. This is based on infants and children having a yang constitution. Infants may have a normal pulse rate of 6 beats per respiration. School children may have a normal rate of 5 beats per respiration. At puberty, the pulse has force. This is because of the maturation of the viscera and bowels and therefore the exuberance of the qi and blood. In old people, the pulse becomes relaxed and weak. This is because of the decline and debility of the viscera and bowels and the concomitant vacuity weakness of the qi and blood.

Sex

A man's pulse has force. A woman's pulse is typically weaker than a man's. During pregnancy, the pulse is usually slippery and rapid. The *Bin Hu Mai Xue (The Lakeside Master's Study of the Pulse)* says that because women are more yin and men more yang and because the right side of the body is yin and the left is yang, it is normal for men's pulses to be larger on the left and women's to be larger on the right. I have not found this to be the case in my clinical practice.

Body Type

Fat people mostly have a deep pulse. Skinny people have comparatively large pulses.

Lifestyle

People who are more athletic and active typically have a relaxed pulse. If the pulse is moderate and relaxed in that it is not wiry, this is a sign of good health. But if it is relaxed to the point that its rate is on the verge of slow, this is not necessarily good. In many athletes, this is a sign of heart qi vacuity due to overtaxation.

Anatomical Variation

A laterally displaced pulse is called a *fan guan mai*, opposite gate pulse. This means that the pulse may be felt not on top of the styloid process but on the side of the forearm. There is also what is called an oblique-running pulse. This describes a radial artery which runs obliquely and not longitudinally. Most commonly, these anatomical anomalies are found on only one wrist. In that case, one only examines the normal wrist. In addition, some patients will have a ganglion cyst at the styloid process which makes pulse examination on that hand impossible. In this case as well, one then only examines the normal pulse on the other hand.

Seasonal Variation

It is axiomatic in Chinese medicine that heaven and humanity correspond to each other (*tian ren xiang ying*). This means that changes in the macrocosm will have their analogues within the microcosm of the human body. In terms of the pulse, this means that the pulse changes throughout the four seasons of spring, summer, autumn, and winter. The chart below shows both the ancient and contemporary terms used to describe these correspondences.

Season	Modern	Ancient
***Chun*, spring**	*Xian*, wiry	*Xian,* wiry
***Xia*, summer**	*Hong*, surging	*Hong*, surging
***Qiu*, autumn**	*Fu*, floating	*Mao*, hair(-like)
***Dong*, winter**	*Chen*, deep	*Shi*, stone(-like)

In theory, it is not necessarily a sign of disease for the pulses to exhibit these images in their corresponding seasons. However, if in the spring there is a wiry pulse and other signs and symptoms of liver depression and qi stagnation, this is not normal and should be treated as a disease pulse and pattern. Likewise, in the fall, if there is a floating, fine, and rapid pulse with a dry sore throat, dry cough, fever, and no or scanty phlegm, this is also not normal and should be treated as a disease pulse and pattern. What this does mean is that if the pulse is a little more floating during the fall or a little wiry during the spring and these changes are not accompanied by any other disease changes and transformations, they should not necessarily be treated as pathological.

It is also normal for everyone to have a somewhat hook-like pulse. This means a pulse which starts off deep in the cubit or *chi* position and then rises to become floating in the *cun* or inch position. In other words, it is not necessarily abnormal for the *cun* position to be relatively floating and the *chi* position to be relatively deep. However, a very pronounced, hook-like pulse indicates counterflow qi surging upward. This usually involves the *chong mai* and, in women, is typically associated with gynecological diseases with concomitant spiritual disquietude.

6
The Indications of the Main Pulse Images

In this chapter, I present the indications of the 27-29 pulses given in several different Chinese sources. The first quote is from Hua Tuo's *Zhong Zang Jing (Classic of the Central Viscera)*. Hua Tuo's birth date is usually given at about 110 CE, so these indications are quite early ones. Nonetheless, these indications are still basically accepted in contemporary TCM pulse examination. The second list is a fairly simple contemporary one. It discusses each of the main pulse images as a single entity. The following two lists discuss more complicated, combined pulse images and their indications. In particular, the fourth list groups the various pulse images into several major categories. It is my experience that going over such lists again and again helps the process of memorization.

If the reader comes across a seeming discrepancy between one of these lists and another, they are recommended to think more deeply about the mechanisms at work in the various pulse images until they can account for these seemingly different points of view. In this way one will get a fuller, rounder understanding of the pulse and its indications, remembering that here in the West a simplistic understanding will fail us when we attempt to treat the chronic, complicated diseases which constitute our main patient population.

Hua Tuo's Indications for the Main Pulse Images

> The pulse is the precursor to qi and blood. When qi and blood are exuberant, the pulse is exuberant. When qi and blood are debilitated, the pulse is debilitated. When qi and blood are hot, the pulse is rapid. When

qi and blood are cold, the pulse is slow. When qi and blood are normal, the pulse is moderate...[1]

Moreover, the various rapid pulses indicate heat; the various slow pulses indicate cold; the various tight pulses indicate pain; the various floating pulses indicate wind; the various slippery pulses indicate vacuity; the various hidden pulses indicate gathering; the various long pulses indicate repletion; and the various short pulses indicate vacuity. Further, all the short, choppy, deep, slow, hidden pulses are ascribed to yin. The rapid, slippery, long, floating, and tight pulses are ascribed to yang.[2]

Contemporary Indications of the Main Discreet Pulse Images

1. ***Fu Mai*, Floating Pulse:** This is characterized as a yang pulse. It is mostly seen in wind evil, external guest, exterior patterns. If floating and forceless, pertains to vacuity patterns.

2. ***Chen Mai*, Deep Pulse:** This is characterized as a yin pulse. It is largely seen in those who have evil qi hidden internally or interior patterns. Also may be seen in qi stagnation or vacuity patterns.

3. ***Chi Mai*, Slow Pulse:** This is characterized as a yin pulse. It is largely seen in internal, viscera, yin, cold patterns. If floating and simultaneously slow, this is yang vacuity externally. If deep and slow, this is fire debility internally.

4. ***Shu Mai*, Rapid Pulse:** This is characterized as a yang pulse. It is usually seen in bowel heat patterns. If floating and rapid with diminished strength, this is a yin vacuity pattern. If deep and rapid with strength, this is a fire heat internally exuberant pattern.

---

[1] Hua Tuo, *Master Hua's Classic of the Central Viscera*, trans. by Yang Shou-zhong, Blue Poppy Press, Boulder, CO, 1993, p. 29

[2] *Ibid.*, p. 29

5. *Hua Mai,* Slippery Pulse: The slippery pulse may be seen in two types of conditions. 1) Blood exuberance leads to a slippery, uninhibited pulse. This is the pulse of pregnancy or a non-disease pulse. 2) Pathologically, this pulse may be seen in phlegm patterns, food accumulation internally stopped, or serious evil qi patterns. Therefore, the slippery pulse may be either a *ping mai* or a *bing mai.*

6. *Se Mai,* Choppy Pulse: This pulse is seen in blood scant or essence damaged conditions. It can also be seen with qi stagnation or cold damp patterns.

7. *Xu Mai,* Vacuous Pulse: This pulse is floating, large, slow, and weak. It is seen in blood vacuity patterns and also damage by summerheat.

8. *Shi Mai,* Replete Pulse: This pulse has force and is long, large, and tight. It is seen in exuberant evils patterns, fire patterns with evils exuberant, or evil repletion gathering and binding.

9. *Chang Mai,* Long Pulse: This pulse is seen in qi counterflow, fire exuberant patterns. It is also a non-disease image.

10. *Duan Mai,* Short Pulse: The short pulse is an image of not reaching. It is also seen in source qi vacuity and debility patterns.

11. *Hong Mai,* Surging Pulse: This pulse is seen in evil exuberant, fire hyperactive patterns. If surging and forceless, this is vacuity surging. It is a manifestation of fire floating and water drying up.

12. *Wei Mai,* Faint Pulse: The faint pulse is seen in collapse of yang patterns, qi and blood great debility. In emergencies, it may show inability to redeem the situation.

13. *Jin Mai,* Tight Pulse: The tight pulse is seen in cold evil patterns and pain patterns.

14. *Huan Mai,* **Moderate (*i.e.,* Retarded) Pulse:** The moderate pulse is typically not a disease pulse. It shows that the pulse has stomach (qi). However, damp evils disease may also manifest a relaxed pulse.

15. *Kou Mai,* **Scallion-stalk Pulse:** This pulse is seen in great blood loss conditions, such as hematemesis, epistaxis, *beng lou* (*i.e.*, flooding and leaking), etc.

16. *Xian Mai,* **Wiry Pulse:** This pulse is seen in liver wind patterns. It is also seen in phlegm rheum and pain patterns.

17. *Ge Mai,* **Drumskin Pulse:** This pulse is large, wiry, and tense. It can be felt superficially but becomes empty on pressure. In other words, the outside is tight but the inside is empty. It is seen in exterior cold extreme exuberance patterns. In males, it may also be seen in essence blood consumption detriment. In females, in miscarriage.

18. *Lao Mai,* **Confined Pulse:** This is large, wiry, and replete but can only be felt deep. It is seen in accumulation and gathering patterns.

19. *Ru Mai,* **Soggy Pulse:** This pulse is fine, soft, and floating. It is seen in yin vacuity patterns. It can also be seen in kidney vacuity, marrow exhausted, and essence damaged (patterns).

20. *Ruo Mai,* **Weak Pulse:** The weak pulse is seen in yang debility patterns. In chronic diseases, it is not always critical.

21. *San Mai,* **Scattered Pulse:** This pulse is seen in kidney qi debility and decay patterns. If one sees the scattered pulse appear during the course of a disease, the patient is doomed to death.

22. *Xi Mai,* **Fine Pulse:** The thready pulse is seen in qi debility patterns. It can also be seen in damp patterns. If seen in either vacuity, taxation or detriment, the disease is serious.

23. ***Fu Mai,*** **Hidden Pulse:** This pulse is seen when disease evils are very deeply located in interior patterns.

24. ***Dong Mai,*** **Stirring Pulse:** This pulse is seen in pain patterns and also in diseases caused by fright.

25. ***Cu Mai,*** **Skipping or Rapid Irregularly Interrupted Pulse:** A skipping pulse is rapid but has one stop. It is seen in fire patterns and also when the qi aspect has a blockage.

26. ***Jie Mai,*** **Bound Pulse:** This pulse is slow and occasionally has one stop. It is seen in accumulation, stagnation, stasis, and obstruction.

27. ***Dai Mai,*** **Regularly Interrupted Pulse:** This is seen in yang qi debility and decay. If seen in the course of a disease, the situation is already critical and the patient is in immanent danger.

28. ***Ji Mai,*** **Racing Pulse:** If one sees a *ji mai* during the course of a disease, this is yang qi extremely exuberant and yin qi on the point of drying up.

Indications of Combined Pulse Images

The following quote from Zhu Dan-xi in his *Ge Zhi Yu Lun (Extra Treatises Based on Investigation & Inquiry)* points out the fact that, although the pulse images must be first learned separately, in clinical practice, they usually present in combinations:

> If the physician intends to determine whether the blood and qi are diseased or not, they have no other way to obtain that knowledge than by palpating the pulse. The pulse can present a number of different images, and the types that are recorded in the *Mai Jing (Pulse Classic)* are twenty plus four [in number], namely, the floating, deep, hollow, slippery, replete, wiry, tight, surging, minute, relaxed, choppy, slow, hidden, soggy, weak, rapid, fine, stirring, vacuous, skipping, bound, regularly

> interrupted, drumskin, and scattered [pulses]. *Usually [more than one of] these images are seen in combination.*[3]

1. *Fu Mai,* Floating Pulse

The floating pulse indicates exterior patterns. It also indicates miscellaneous diseases due to blood vacuity. Further, it indicates vacuity detriment of yang qi floating to the outside. A floating and slow pulse indicates exterior wind. A floating and rapid pulse indicates exterior heat. A floating and tight pulse indicates exterior cold. A floating pulse with strength indicates exterior repletion. A floating pulse without strength indicates exterior vacuity.

2. *Chen Mai,* Deep Pulse

A deep pulse indicates interior patterns. A deep, rapid pulse indicates interior heat. A deep, slow pulse indicates interior cold. A deep, slippery pulse indicates phlegm rheum. A deep pulse with strength indicates interior repletion patterns and also accumulation and stagnation, cold congelation, etc. A deep, forceless pulse indicates interior vacuity patterns, mostly yang qi vacuity and debility.

3. *Chi Mai,* Slow Pulse

A slow pulse indicates cold patterns. It also indicates concretions and conglomerations, accumulations and gatherings. A slow, forceful pulse indicates chilly pain patterns. A slow, forceless pulse indicates vacuity cold patterns. A slow, weak pulse indicates yang vacuity and yin exuberance. A slow, slippery pulse indicates cold phlegm.

---

[3] Zhu Dan-xi, *Extra Treatises Based on Investigation & Inquiry*, trans. by Yang Shou-zhong & Duan Wu-jin, Blue Poppy, Press Boulder, CO, 1994, p. 13, italics added by Bob Flaws.

4. *Shu Mai,* Rapid Pulse

A rapid pulse indicates heat patterns. A floating, rapid pulse indicates exterior heat. A deep, rapid pulse indicates interior heat. A rapid, forceful pulse indicates replete heat patterns. A rapid, forceless pulse indicates vacuity heat patterns. A rapid, fine, and soft pulse indicates yin vacuity, internal heat. A rapid, large, forceless pulse indicates vacuous yang floating to the outside.

5. *Xu Mai,* Vacuous Pulse

A vacuous pulse indicates vacuity patterns. It mainly essentially indicates qi and blood vacuity, damage by summerheat, yin vacuity fever, essence deficiency and scanty blood, etc.

6. *Shi Mai,* Replete Pulse

A replete pulse indicates repletion patterns. It essentially indicates replete fire overwhelming and exuberant, and qi and blood stasis and binding. A replete pulse also indicates food accumulation, constipation due to bound heat in the stomach and intestines, qi pain, yang toxins, vomiting, mania, delirious speech, and other such patterns.

7. *Kou Mai,* Scallion-stalk Pulse

A scallion-stalk pulse indicates pathoconditions with loss of blood. Such loss of blood pathoconditions include vomiting of blood, hematuria, bloody dysentery, bloody stools, and women's flooding and leaking (*i.e.*, menometrorrhagia) when the loss of blood is severe.

8. *Xian Mai,* Wiry Pulse

A wiry pulse indicates liver/gallbladder diseases. It also indicates phlegm rheum, chronic cold, and pain patterns. A wiry, large, and slippery pulse indicates yang patterns. A wiry, tight, and fine pulse indicates yin patterns. A wiry, floating pulse indicates branch rheum. A wiry, deep pulse indicates suspended rheum. A wiry, rapid pulse indicates extreme heat. A wiry, slow pulse indicates exuberant cold. A wiry, large pulse indicates vacuity detriment. A wiry, small pulse indicates hypertonicity. If one hand is wiry, this mostly indicates rheum elusive mass. If both hands are wiry, this mostly indicates chronic cold. A wiry, hard pulse indicates a serious disease. A wiry, soft pulse indicates a light disease.

9. *Hong Mai,* Surging Pulse

A surging pulse indicates diseases with intense heat. Most often, a surging pulse appears with a rapid pulse, in which case it indicates heart fire flaming upward, heat congesting in the lungs, intense heat in the *yang ming*, liver yang exuberance, kidney vacuity yin fire, yin vacuity diarrhea and dysentery, etc.

10. *Wei Mai,* Faint Pulse

The faint pulse indicates diseases with qi and blood vacuity. It can also indicate lung qi vacuity, heart yang vacuity, spleen/stomach qi vacuity, kidney source vacuity detriment, etc. The faint pulse mostly corresponds diagnostically to vacuity detriment of the viscera and bowels.

11. *Hua Mai,* Slippery Pulse

The slippery pulse indicates phlegm rheum, long-standing food, vomiting, acid regurgitation, a stiff tongue, coughing, liver heat, wasting thirst, dysentery, *tui shan*, and strangury patterns. It also indicates women's diseases due to qi and blood deficiency and detriment after curettage of the uterus or postpartum.

The slippery pulse is commonly seen in women during pregnancy. It is also a pulse indicative of a normal physiology as long as it is not combined with any other of these disease pulses.

12. *Se Mai,* Choppy Pulse

The choppy pulse indicates blood vacuity, essence debility, qi stagnation, blood stasis, yin collapse, and other such diseases. The choppy pulse can also indicate chest *bi*, spleen/stomach vacuity weakness, stomach reflux, essence blood dual vacuity constipation, strangury patterns, intestinal wind with descending blood, blood loss, spermatorrhea, and vacuity diarrhea. It can also indicate wind stroke with hemiplegia, concretions and conglomerations, etc.

13. *Jin Mai,* Tight Pulse

The tight pulse indicates cold patterns. A tight, floating pulse indicates exterior cold. A tight, deep pulse indicates interior cold. A tight pulse mostly indicates lung cold wheezing and cough, liver cold wind *xian*, spleen cold vomiting of chilly phlegm, and cold evils resulting in pain patterns.

14. *Huan Mai,* Relaxed or Moderate Pulse

The relaxed pulse indicates wind patterns, damp patterns, and spleen vacuity patterns. A relaxed, floating pulse indicates wind stroke exterior vacuity. A relaxed, deep pulse indicates damp stagnation of the channels and network vessels. A relaxed, fine, and slow pulse indicates spleen/stomach vacuity weakness. A relaxed pulse mostly indicates concretions and conglomerations, torticollis, dizziness and vertigo, moist diarrhea, wind *bi*, lower extremity atony and flaccidity, and other such patterns.

15. *Fu Mai,* Hidden Pulse

The hidden pulse indicates depression and binding of evils in the interior, obstruction and blockage of the channels and vessels, and qi and blood stasis and stagnation. It also indicates accumulation of food, accumulation of rheum, old phlegm, and acute vomiting and diarrhea.

16. *Xi Mai,* Fine Pulse

The fine pulse indicates internal damage vacuity taxation and yin and yang dual vacuity. It also indicates qi and blood dual vacuity, taxation detriment of the seven affects, low back kidney disease, spontaneous sweating, etc.

17. *Jie Mai,* Bound Pulse

The knotted pulse indicates yang vacuity, yin exuberance. It also indicates qi stagnation and blood stasis, old phlegm binding and stagnating, accumulations and gatherings, concretions and conglomerations, *shan* qi, *yong* swelling, and other such patterns.

18. *Ruo Mai,* Weak Pulse

The weak pulse indicates yin and yang dual vacuity and yang qi vacuity and debility. Bone atony, sinew atony, palpitations, spontaneous sweating, and shortness of breath due to exhaustion affecting various viscera and bowels causing yang qi vacuity and debility, lower burner yin essence extreme deficiency and detriment, and other such patterns typically present a weak pulse.

19. *Ruan Mai,* Soft Pulse (also called a *Ru Mai,* Soggy Pulse)

A soft pulse indicates yin vacuity, blood vacuity, and damp diseases. It also indicates yang vacuity spontaneous sweating and central qi insufficiency. Sea of marrow emptiness and vacuity, construction and blood vacuity scantness, yin vacuity thief (*i.e.*, night) sweats, damage of both the essence and blood, bone steaming and tidal fever, flooding and leaking, spleen dampness moist diarrhea, etc., commonly manifest a soft pulse.

20. *Dai Mai,* Regularly Interrupted Pulse

A regularly interrupted pulse indicates visceral qi vacuity and debility and source yang insufficiency. It also indicates wind patterns, pain patterns, the seven affects and fear and fright, falling and tumbling detriment and damage, etc. Spleen/stomach qi vacuity with vomiting and diarrhea, yang vacuity abdominal pain, diarrhea and dysentery, and other such patterns can also commonly manifest a regularly interrupted pulse.

Combined Pulse Images & Their Indications Grouped According to Categories

Floating Pulses

1. *Fu Mai,* Floating Pulse

Main diseases: A floating pulse mainly indicates exterior patterns. If it has force, this is exterior repletion. If without force, this is exterior vacuity. If floating and tight, wind cold. If floating and rapid, wind heat. If floating and relaxed, wind damp. If floating and slow, wind vacuity. If floating and vacuous, summerheat exhaustion. If floating and scallion-stalk, loss of blood. If floating and surging, vacuity heat. If floating and soggy, yin vacuity. If floating and choppy, blood damage. If floating and short, qi disease. If floating and wiry, phlegm rheum. If floating and slippery, phlegm heat. *In chronic disease, this pulse is associated with counterflow patterns.*

2. *Hong Mai,* Surging Pulse

Main diseases: A surging pulse mainly indicates heat patterns. Also rules yin vacuity, yang exuberance. If it has force, the disease moves forward. If it is without force, this is righteous vacuity.

3. *Kou Mai,* Scallion-stalk Pulse

Main diseases: A scallion-stalk pulse mainly indicates desertion of blood and collapse of yin.

4. *Ge Mai,* Drumskin Pulse

Main diseases: A drumskin pulse mainly indicates loss of blood. It also mainly indicates vacuity cold. In males, essence blood insufficiency. In females, half delivery (*i.e.*, miscarriage) or flooding precipitation (*i.e.*, profuse uterine bleeding).

5. *Ru Mai,* Soggy Pulse

Main diseases: A soggy pulse mainly indicates qi and blood insufficiency over time causing dampness, or *vice versa*. Spontaneous sweating, diarrhea, and diminished appetite.

6. *Xu Mai,* Vacuous Pulse

Main diseases: This pulse mainly indicates qi and blood insufficiency. Also damage by summerheat and sudden, violent desertion.

Deep Pulses

7. *Chen Mai,* Deep Pulse

Main diseases: The deep pulse mainly indicates interior pattems. Without strength, interior vacuity. With strength, interior repletion. Deep and slow, inveterate chill. Deep and rapid, internal heat. Deep and choppy, blood binding. Deep and weak, vacuity and debility. Deep and confined, hard accumulations. Deep and tight, chilly ache. Deep and relaxed/retarded, cold dampness. Deep and fine, scant qi. Deep and wiry, elusive mass pain.

8. *Fu Mai,* Hidden Pulse

Main diseases: This pulse mainly indicates yang qi debility and diminution. It also rules yin patterns with aching and pain. If all six pulses are deep and hidden, the four limbs experience inversion chill.

9. *Lao Mai,* Confined Pulse

Main diseases: The confined pulse mainly indicates interior patterns. It also mainly indicates wind epilepsy, inflexibility, and cramping, hard accumulations internally hidden, and running piglet (*ben tun*), sudden, violent counterflow.

10. *Ruo Mai,* Weak Pulse

Main diseases: The weak pulse rules qi and blood insufficiency. After disease, the righteous may be vacuous. In this case, a weak pulse is normal. However, if during a disease due to evil repletion one sees a weak pulse, this is an ominous sign.

Slow Pulses

11. *Chi Mai,* Slow Pulse

Main diseases: The slow pulse mainly indicates viscera cold. Also mainly indicates yang vacuity. With strength, chilly pain. Without strength, vacuity cold. Floating and slow, exterior cold. Deep and slow, interior cold. Slow and choppy, blood disease. Slow and slippery, qi disease with scant qi (shortness of breath) and heart disease.

12. *Huan Mai,* Relaxed (*i.e.*, Retarded) Pulse

Main diseases: It is essential to see this pulse at the right *guan* (where it is normal. This means that the pulse is not wiry). As a *bing mai*, this pulse rules diseases which require comparative examination with other simultaneously appearing pulse images. If floating and relaxed, damage by wind. If deep and relaxed, damp disease. If relaxed and large, liver wind internally exuberant. If relaxed and weak, heart qi insufficiency.

13. *Se Mai,* Choppy Pulse

Main diseases: The choppy pulse mainly indicates scant blood and damaged essence, blood stasis and qi stagnation. It also mainly indicates heart diseases and palpitations.

Rapid Pulses

14. *Shu Mai,* Rapid Pulse

Main diseases: This pulse mainly indicates heat. It also rules vacuity. With strength, repletion. Without strength, vacuity.

15. *Hua Mai,* Slippery Pulse

Main diseases: This pulse mainly indicates repletion and it also mainly indicates heat. It mainly indicates phlegm and food (stagnation). Floating and slippery, wind illness. Deep and slippery, phlegm, food. Slippery and rapid, phlegm fire. Slippery with harmonious beat (*chong he*), stomach qi or pregnancy.

16. *Dong Mai,* Stirring Pulse

Main diseases: This pulse mainly indicates fright palpitations. It also mainly indicates aching, pain, and fever.

17. *Ji Mai,* Racing Pulse

Main diseases: This pulse mainly indicates heat and also mainly indicates heart palpitations.

Short Pulses

18. *Duan Mai,* Short Pulse

Main diseases: This pulse mainly indicates qi and blood vacuity detriment.

19. *Wei Mai,* Faint Pulse

Main diseases: The faint pulse mainly indicates qi desertion and essence consumption, yang minute and yin weak.

20. *Xi Mai,* Fine Pulse

Main diseases: This pulse mainly indicates all types of vacuity and insufficiency. Fine and rapid, yin vacuity with internal heat.

Long Pulses

21. *Chang Mai,* Long Pulse

Main diseases: This pulse mainly indicates surplus, qi counterflow, and fire exuberance. One must compare it to other patterns appearing in the body.

22. *Xian Mai,* Wiry Pulse

Main diseases: The wiry pulse mainly indicates liver wind. It also mainly indicates pain, malaria-like diseases, and phlegm rheum. Wiry and rapid, much heat. Wiry and slow, much cold. Yang wiry, (*i.e.*, inch wiry) headache. Yin wiry, (*i.e.*, cubit wiry) abdominal pain. One side wiry, rheum elusive mass. Both sides wiry, recalcitrant, inveterate cold.

23. *Jin Mai,* Tight Pulse

Main diseases: This pulse mainly indicates cold evils. It also mainly indicates all sorts of pain. Floating and tight, in the exterior. Deep and tight, in the interior.

24. *Shi Mai,* Replete Pulse

Main diseases: The replete pulse mainly indicates evil exuberance having a surplus. It mainly indicates large evils, great accumulations, great gatherings. If in diarrhea one sees a replete pulse, this is a counterflow pattern. If in a vacuity pattern one sees a replete pulse, this portends a poor prognosis.

Interrupted Pulses

25. *San Mai,* Scattered Pulse

Main diseases: This pulse mainly indicates qi and blood consumed and scattered. The visceral qi is on the verge of exhaustion. It also mainly indicates heart qi insufficiency and heart palpitations.

26. *Jie Mai,* Bound Pulse

Main diseases: This pulse mainly indicates heart palpitations.

27. *Cu Mai,* Skipping or Rapid Irregularly Interrupted Pulse

Main diseases: This pulse mainly indicates replete heat. It also mainly indicates righteous debility and wheezing and cough.

28. *Dai Mai,* Regularly Interrupted Pulse

Main diseases: This pulse mainly indicates fright palpitations and qi chaos. It also mainly indicates visceral qi debility and diminution.

Signs & Symptoms Corroborating the Pulse

As stated in the Introduction, in TCM, no one sign or symptom always means any one thing. What a sign or a symptom means in a given patient is always determined by the constellation of other signs and symptoms with which it appears. The list below, therefore, gives corroborating signs and symptoms for various of the indications of the main pulse images. If one assigns a certain meaning to a particular pulse image but then cannot substantiate that hypothesis by the presence of the typical corroborating signs and symptoms, then the practitioner knows they need to think again about their interpretation of the pulse.

1. *Fu Mai,* Floating Pulse

When a floating pulse indicates an exterior pattern, the corroborating symptoms will be a short disease course, dislike of cold, fever, headache, body pain, stiff neck, stuffed nose, cough, wheezing, a thin, white tongue coating, etc.

2. *Chi Mai,* Slow Pulse

When a slow pulse indicates a cold pattern, the corroborating symptoms are dislike of cold, a somber, white facial complexion, loose stools, clear, long urination, a pale tongue with a white, moist coating, etc.

3. *Shu Mai,* Rapid Pulse

A rapid pulse indicates heat patterns. The corroborating symptoms of heat are fever, thirst, a red face, red lips, constipation, a red tongue with a yellow coating, etc.

4. *Xu Mai,* Vacuous Pulse; *Xi Mai,* Fine Pulse; *Ruan Mai,* Soft Pulse; *Ruo Mai,* Weak Pulse

All these pulses indicate vacuity patterns. Vacuity is corroborated by spiritual exhaustion, lack of strength, bodily fatigue, a faded, white facial color, an emaciated body, weak breathing and sluggish speech, heart palpitations, shortness of breath, loss of sleep, poor memory, spontaneous sweating, night sweats, spermatorrhea, urinary incontinence, aching and pain which desires pressure, a pale tongue with no or scant coating, etc.

5. *Shi Mai,* Replete Pulse

A replete pulse indicates repletion patterns. These are corroborated by symptoms such as essence spirit hyperactivity and vigor, a high (*i.e.*, loud), husky voice, chest and abdominal distention and fullness, aching and pain resisting pressure, constipation, tenesmus, inhabited urination, a thick, slimy coating, etc.

6. *Fu Jin Mai,* Floating, Tight Pulse

A floating, tight pulse indicates exterior cold patterns. Corroborating signs and symptoms include dislike of cold, fever, no sweating, headache, stiff neck, joint aching and pain, a thin, white tongue coating, etc.

7. *Fu Huan Mai,* Floating, Relaxed Pulse

A floating, relaxed pulse indicates exterior vacuity patterns. Corroborating signs and symptoms include fever, dislike of wind, stuffy nose, spontaneous sweating, a pale tongue with a white coating, etc.

8. *Fu Shu Mai,* Floating, Rapid Pulse

A floating, rapid pulse indicates an exterior heat pattern. Corroborating signs and symptoms include fever, slight dislike of cold, thirst, yellow urine, slight sweating, a thin, yellow tongue coating, etc.

9. *Chen Chi Mai,* Deep, Slow Pulse

A deep, slow pulse indicates interior cold patterns. Corroborating signs and symptoms include bodily cold, chilled extremities, a somber, white facial complexion, no thirst or thirst with a desire for hot drinks, thin, watery phlegm, loose stools, long, clear urination, a pale tongue with a white, glossy coating, etc.

10. *Chen Shu Mai,* Deep, Rapid Pulse

A deep, rapid pulse indicates interior heat patterns. Corroborating signs and symptoms include a flushed red face, heart vexation, thirst, yellow, sticky phlegm, constipation, short, scant, reddish yellow urination, a red tongue with a yellow coating, etc.

11. *Ruo Mai,* Weak Pulse

A weak pulse indicates vacuity patterns. Corroborating signs and symptoms include weak qi and sluggish speech, reduced appetite, bodily fatigue, dizziness, heart palpitations, a pale, tender tongue with a thin, white coating, etc.

12. *Chen Shi Mai,* Deep, Replete Pulse

A deep, replete pulse indicates interior repletion patterns. Corroborating signs and symptoms include chest and abdominal distention and fullness, aching and pain which resists pressure, constipation, a yellow, slimy tongue coating, etc.

13. *Xi Shu Mai,* Fine, Rapid Pulse

A fine, rapid pulse indicates yin vacuity patterns. Corroborating signs and symptoms include afternoon tidal fever, both cheeks flushed red, heat in the centers of the hands and feet (or heat in the hands, feet, and heart), heart vexation and loss of sleep, dizziness and vertigo, a dry mouth and throat, night sweats, dry, bound stools, short, yellow urination, a red tongue with scant coating, etc.

14. *Ruo Mai,* Weak Pulse

A weak pulse indicates yang vacuity patterns. Corroborating signs and symptoms include bodily cold with chilled extremities, a dim (or dusky), pale face, fatigued spirit, lack of strength, spontaneous sweating, no thirst, loose stools, long, clear urination, a pale tongue with a white coating, etc.

15. *Xu Mai,* Vacuous Pulse

A vacuous pulse indicates qi vacuity patterns. Corroborating signs and symptoms include shortness of breath, sluggish speech, bodily fatigue, lack of strength, dizziness and vertigo, a pale tongue with a thin coating, etc.

16. *Xi Mai,* Fine Pulse

A fine pulse indicates blood vacuity patterns. Corroborating signs and symptoms include a pale, white face without luster or a sallow, yellow color, pale, white lips, dizziness and blurred vision, heart palpitations, loss of sleep, numbness of the hands and feet, a pale tongue, etc.

7
Pattern Discrimination & the Pulse Images

TCM as a style bases its treatments on pattern discrimination. In TCM, there are 10 methods of discriminating patterns. These are:

1. Eight principles pattern discrimination (*ba gang bian zheng*)
2. Five phase pattern discrimination (*wu xing bian zheng*)
3. Qi & blood pattern discrimination (*qi xue bian zheng*)
4. Fluids & humors pattern discrimination (*jin ye bian zheng*)
5. Viscera & bowel pattern discrimination (*zang fu bian zheng*)
6. Channel & network vessel pattern discrimination (*jing luo bian zheng*)
7. Disease cause pattern discrimination (*bing yin bian zheng*)
8. Six aspect pattern discrimination (*liu fen bian zheng*)
9. Four aspect pattern discrimination (*si fen bian zheng*)
10. Three burners pattern discrimination (*san jiao bian zheng*)

Below are charts showing the relationships between several of these methods of discriminating patterns and the most common main pulse images associated with those patterns.

Eight Principles Pattern Discrimination & the Pulse

Pattern	Pulse	Pattern	Pulse
Exterior	Floating	**Interior cold**	Deep, slow
Interior	Deep	**Interior heat**	Deep, rapid
Cold	Slow	**Interior vacuity**	Weak
Heat	Rapid	**Interior repletion**	Deep, replete
Vacuity	Vacuous, fine, soft, weak	**Yin vacuity**	Fine, rapid
Repletion	Replete	**Yang vacuity**	Weak
Exterior cold	Floating, tight	**Qi vacuity**	Vacuous, weak
Exterior vacuity	Floating, relaxed	**Blood vacuity**	Fine
Exterior heat	Floating, rapid	**Yin collapse**	Fine, rapid, soft
Exterior repletion	Floating, tight	**Yang collapse**	Minute, weak

Qi & Blood Pattern Discrimination & the Pulse

Pattern	Pulse	Pattern	Pulse
Qi vacuity	Vacuous	**Blood vacuity**	Fine
Qi fall	Vacuous	**Blood stasis**	Fine, slow, choppy
Qi stagnation	Slippery, replete	**Blood heat**	Rapid
Qi counterflow	Wiry, slippery		

Six Aspect Pattern Discrimination & the Pulse

Pattern	Pulse	Pattern	Pulse
Tai yang **exterior vacuity**	Floating, relaxed	***Shao yang*** **(½ inside, ½ outside)**	Floating, wiry
Tai yang **exterior**	Floating, tight	**Spleen yang repletion**	Deep, relaxed, weak
Tai yang **amassing water**	Floating	***Shao yin*** **cold debility transformation**	Deep, minute
Tai yang **amassing blood**	Deep, choppy	***Shao yin*** **heat transformation**	Deep, minute, fine, rapid
Heat scorching the ***yang ming***	Surging	***Jue yin*** **roundworm inversion**	Deep, minute, hidden
Yang ming **bowel repletion**	Deep, replete	**Cold inversion, dry throat, headache**	Deep, wiry, fine

Defensive, Qi, Constructive & Blood Pattern Discrimination & the Pulse

Pattern	Pulse	Pattern	Pulse
Warmth & heat raid the exterior	Floating, rapid	**Heat damages constructive yin**	Rapid, fine
Heat congesting in the lungs	Rapid	**Heat entering the pericardium**	Rapid
Heat depression in the chest & diaphragm	Floating, slippery & rapid	**Blood heat moving recklessly**	Rapid
Intense heat in the *yang ming*	Surging	**Qi & blood both scorched**	Rapid
Heat binding in the intestinal tract	Deep, replete	**Damaged yin, stirring wind**	Rapid, soft (soggy)
Damp heat smoldering & binding in the three heaters	Soggy, rapid		

Viscera & Bowel Pattern Discrimination & the Pulse

Pattern	Pulse	Pattern	Pulse
Heart fire flaming upward	Rapid	**Stomach yin insufficiency**	Fine, rapid
Phlegm fire harassing the heart	Slippery, rapid	**Spleen qi vacuous & weak**	Relaxed, weak, or soggy
Heart blood stasis & accumulation	Bound, regularly interrupted	**Spleen qi fallen down**	Weak, vacuous
Small intestine qi pain	Deep, wiry	**Spleen/stomach vacuity cold**	Deep, slow
Heart yin vacuity	Fine, rapid	**Spleen not containing the blood**	Weak or scallion-stalk
Heart yang vacuity	Fine, weak, bound, or regularly interrupted	**Wind cold fettering the lungs**	Floating, tight
Heart qi vacuity	Fine, weak	**Wind heat attacking the lungs**	Floating, rapid
Heart blood vacuity	Fine soft, weak	**Phlegm heat congesting in the lungs**	Slippery, rapid
Liver blood insufficiency	Wiry, fine	**Phlegm turbidity obstructing the lungs**	Slippery
Liver fire flaming upward	Wiry, rapid	**Large intestine damp heat**	Slippery, rapid
Liver/gallbladder damp heat	Wiry, rapid	**Lung qi vacuity**	Vacuous, weak

Pattern	Pulse	Pattern	Pulse
Liver qi depression & binding	Wiry	**Lung yin vacuity**	Rapid, fine
Liver yang transforming wind	Wiry, rapid	**Large intestine fluid depletion**	Fine
Extreme heat engenders wind	Wiry, rapid	**Intestinal vacuity, slippery desertion**	Weak
Blood vacuity engenders wind	Wiry, fine	**Bladder damp heat**	Slippery, rapid
Cold stagnation in the liver vessel	Deep, wiry	**Kidney yang vacuity**	Deep, weak, slow
Gallbladder depression, phlegm harassing	Wiry	**Kidney yin vacuity**	Fine, rapid
Flourishing of intense stomach fire	Slippery, rapid	**Kidney not grasping the qi**	Vacuous
Food stagnation in the stomach	Slippery	**Kidney essence insufficiency**	Fine, rapid
Spleen/stomach damp heat	Rapid, soggy	**Kidney qi not securing**	Deep, weak
Damp heat confined in the spleen	Soggy, fine		

8
Pulse Images & the Three Positions

So far we have only been talking about the meanings of pulse images in general, irrespective of where these images appear in the pulse. As stated above, the pulse is divided into three sections, in terms of length, which correspond in general to the three burners: *cun* = upper burner, *guan* = middle burner, *chi* = lower burner. Further, each of these three positions corresponds especially to certain of the viscera and bowels located in each of those three burners, for example: right *cun* = lungs, left *cun* = heart. It is possible and even common that different pulse images may be felt in different of these three positions on the two hands.

For instance, there are 27-29 main pulse images. These pulse images often combine to create complicated pulse images. Further, many of these pulse images may appear at different levels of any of 6 basic positions. This means that there are a very large number of possible different pulse readings. It is this very large number of possible combined pulse images which enables Chinese pulse examination to account for the wide variability of disease mechanisms and patterns in individual human beings.

When interpreting the pulse, it is important to identify not only the main overall pulse image or images but also to examine each pulse position on both hands. If there are different pulse images in different positions, their meaning or indications should be interpreted in the light of these positions' anatomical and visceral correspondences. Below are both premodern and contemporary indications for the main pulse images when they occur in the three positions on the two hands. The premodern indications come from the *Bin Hu Mai Xue (The Lakeside Master's Study of the Pulse)*. The main pulse images which are not discussed below in either premodern or contemporary sources are not discussed because they are images which do not manifest only on a single position, such as the interrupted pulses and the racing pulse.

1. *Fu Mai*, Floating Pulse

	Bin Hu Mai Xue	Left	Right
Cun	Headache and vertigo engendered by wind or wind phlegm gathering in the chest	Damage due to wind, fever, headache, vertigo	Common cold, wind evils, cough, excessive phlegm, chest fullness, shortness of breath
Guan	Earth debilitated and liver effulgent	Epigastric fullness, lateral, costal distention, nausea, disgust with food, vexation, oppression	abdominal distention, epigastric fullness, inability to eat, heartburn, stomach pain
Chi	Urine and feces not flowing freely	Bladder wind heat, urination red, astringent, strangurious, painful lower limb swelling & pain	Turbid strangury, hemafecia, joints swollen & painful, wind heat lodged in the lower burner

2. *Chen Mai,* Deep Pulse

	Bin Hu Mai Xue	Left	Right
Cun	Phlegm is depressed and water stopped within the chest	Chest region cold phlegm, qi congestion, chest fullness, heart palpitations, shortness of breath, chest pain, dizziness	Lung cold, stoppage of rheum, chest fullness, chest pain, cough & panting (*i.e.*, asthma), shortness of breath, insufficient respiration
Guan	Cold in the center causing pain due to lack of free flow	Liver depression, lateral costal pain, epigastric distention, abdominal fullness, scanty appetite, heart vexation, a tendency to get angry	Accumulation & stagnation within the stomach, epigastric fullness, abdominal distention, torpid intake, stomachache
Chi	Kidney vacuity affecting the low back and reaching the lower origin	Kidney cold, low back pain, urinary frequency & turbidity, lower abdominal distention & fullness	Low back *bi*, *shan* pain, lower abdomen not smoothly flowing, lower abdominal distention

3. *Chi Mai,* Slow Pulse

	Bin Hu Mai Xue	Left	Right
Cun	Upper burner cold	Cold *bi*, fullness & pain within the chest, devitalized spirit	Lung qi cold and chilled, chest oppression and pain, phlegm stagnation, shortness of breath, simultaneous cough counterflow
Guan	Middle cold pain which is unendurable	Limbs and body inflexible & tense, epigastric fullness, lateral costal distention, heart vexation and oppression	Spleen cold, stomach chilled, food not transformed, accumulation, stagnation, lack of movement
Chi	Kidney vacuity causing heaviness in the low back and legs, urinary incontinence, or unbearable *shan*	Kidney vacuity, diarrhea, low back soreness & pain, no menstruation in women	Abdominal distention & pain, low back soreness, diarrhea

4. *Shu Mai,* Rapid Pulse

	Bin Hu Mai Xue	Left	Right
Cun	Sores in the throat, mouth, and tongue, vomiting red, coughing, lung *yong*	Upper burner headache, sore throat, sores on the mouth & tongue	Cough, spitting blood, panting counterflow, shortness of breath
Guan	Liver fire, stomach fire	Liver heat, red eyes, vexation & fullness, lateral costal pain	Stomach heat, acid regurgitation, heartburn, nausea, abdominal pain, torpid intake
Chi	Fire blazing due to yin vacuity	Dry stools, abdominal distention, red urine, strangury & pain	Bloody stools, turbid strangury, spermatorrhea, low back pain

5. *Hua Mai,* Slippery Pulse

	Bin Hu Mai Xue	Left	Right
Cun	Phlegm in the diaphragm engendering vomiting, acid regurgitation, stiff tongue, cough	Heart vexation & heat, dizziness, heart palpitations, shortness of breath, loss of sleep, excessive dreams	Cough, excessive phlegm, panting counterflow, shortness of breath
Guan	Lodged food, liver/spleen heat	Headache, vertigo, lateral costal distention and pain, heart vexation, tendency to get angry, scanty appetite, epigastric oppression	Epigastric fullness, abdominal distention, food already eaten not transformed
Chi	Thirst, dysentery, *shan*, strangury	Low back pain	Strangury & pain, hematuria, red, astringent urination, lower limb swelling & pain

6. *Se Mai*, Choppy Pulse

	Bin Hu Mai Xue	Left	Right
Cun	Heart vacuity pain in the chest	Heart palpitations, shortness of breath, heart pain, racing heart	Upper burner chilly glomus, shortness of breath, upper arm pain, vacuity cough, spontaneous perspiration
Guan	Stomach vacuity, lateral costal distention	Liver vacuity, blood scanty, chest & lateral costal distention & pain, heart vexation, a tendency to get angry, epigastric fullness, no thought for food	Dry stools, fluid consumption
Chi	Damaged essence and blood in the lower burner causing knotting in the intestines, urinary strangury, or hemafecia	Damaged essence, menstrual irregularity, lower abdominal distention & pain	Abdominal cold, chilled feet

7. *Xu Mai,* Vacuous Pulse

	Bin Hu Mai Xue	Left	Right
Cun	Blood not nourishing the heart	Heart palpitations, shortness of breath, fright palpitations, dizziness, tinnitus, chest oppression, heart vexation & heat	Spontaneous perspiration, cough & panting, shortness of breath, insufficient respiration, vacuity cough, facial complexion a somber white
Guan	Abdominal distention, food not digested	Blood vacuity not constructing, lateral costal distention, pain, & discomfort, heart vexation, a tendency to get angry, devitalized eating & drinking, dizziness, vertigo	Spleen vacuity, scanty appetite, epigastric fullness, abdominal distention, sluggish distention, superficial edema, loose stools
Chi	Damaged essence and blood, *bi* & atony, bone steaming	Low back soreness, leg pain, lower limb atony, *bi,* insensitivity, spermatorrhea, daybreak diarrhea, menstrual irregularity	Scanty appetite, loose stools, clear, long urination, lower abdominal distention & pain, spermatorrhea, menstrual irregularity

8. *Shi Mai,* Replete Pulse

	Bin Hu Mai Xue	Left	Right
Cun	Replete wind heat in the head causing sore throat, stiff tongue, chest fullness	Sores in the mouth & tongue, sore throat, heart vexation & heat, red tongue, heart palpitations, qi congestion, stiff tongue, head dizziness & pain	Shortness of breath, chest fullness, throat dry & painful, cough counterflow, hasty panting, the presence of phlegm
Guan	Spleen heat and abdominal fullness	Epigastric & lateral costal distention & pain, disgust for food, heart vexation, tendency to get angry, head dizziness & pain	Epigastric distention, stomachache, scanty appetite, heartburn, a red tongue with a shiny, yellow coating
Chi	Repletion in the low back and intestines with pain due to lack of free flow	Red, astringent, painful urination, urinary strangury, lower limb swelling & pain, constipation	Lower abdominal distention & pain, short, red urination, blocked menstruation, excessive vaginal discharge, non-smoothly flowing stools or dry, parched stools

9. *Hong Mai,* Surging Pulse

	Bin Hu Mai Xue	Left	Right
Cun	Left: Surging heart fire flames up to the upper burner. Right: Metal cannot endure the lung vessel's surging	Bitter taste in the mouth, heart heat, heart vexation, vertigo, red eyes, mouth ulcers, headache	Lung heat, chest distention & pain, cough, panting counterflow, shortness of breath, excessive phlegm, sore throat
Guan	Liver fire and stomach vacuity	Liver heat, abdominal distention, lateral costal fullness & pain, dizziness & vertigo, heart vexation, tendency to get angry, loss of sleep, red eyes	Stomach heat, epigastric pain, heartburn, clamoring stomach, nausea, vomiting, scanty appetite, torpid intake
Chi	Kidney vacuity, yin fire	Turbid strangury, red, astringent urination, low back pain, lower limb swelling & pain	Lower abdominal distention & fullness, low back soreness, dry stools, hematuria, turbid strangury

10. *Wei Mai,* Faint Pulse

	Bin Hu Mai Xue	Left	Right
Cun	Rapid breathing, heart palpitations	Heart qi insufficiency, lung vacuity, qi weakness	Chest cold, glomus & pain, chilly phlegm congelation & binding
Guan	Distention and fullness	Lateral costal fullness, cold limbs, inflexibility & cramping of the hands & feet	Spleen vacuity, abdominal distention, scanty appetite, fatigue, abdominal pain
Chi	Essence and blood weakness, aversion to cold, thirsting and wasting, *bi* pain	Damaged essence in males, uterine bleeding in females	Lower abdominal distention and fullness, chilly pain below the navel

11. *Jin Mai*, Tight Pulse

	Bin Hu Mai Xue	Left	Right
Cun	Left: Cold evils in the exterior. Right: Damage by internal cold evils	Head dizziness & pain, chest oppression, qi not soothed	Stuffed nose, chest oppression, shortness of breath, cough with spitting up of chilly phlegm
Guan	Heart and abdominal pain and heaviness	Lateral costal pain, abdominal distention, sinews contracted, inflexible & tense	Stomach & epigastric distention & pain, hiccup
Chi	Yin chill causing running piglet and *shan pain*	Low back pain, leg soreness, lower abdominal pain	Distention & pain below the navel, lower abdominal cold *shan*

12. *Huan Mai,* Relaxed Pulse

	Bin Hu Mai Xue	Left	Right
Cun	Wind evils causing upper back and neck stiffness	*Shao yin* blood vacuity, heart palpitations, heart fluster, loss of sleep, excessive dreams	Floating & relaxed; attack of wind evils
Guan	Left: Wind vertigo. Right: Stomach vacuity	Liver wind internally stirring	Deep & relaxed; torpid intake, abdominal distention, spleen weakness, damp invasion
Chi	Watery diarrhea when relaxed and soft. Wind constipation when relaxed and choppy. No strength in lower limbs, difficult movement when relaxed and weak	Dizziness, tinnitus, spermatorrhea, low back & knee soreness & weakness	Relaxed & fine; debility of true yang

13. *Kou Mai*, Scallion-stalk Pulse

	Bin Hu Mai Xue	Left	Right
Cun	Accumulated blood in the chest	Heart blood reckless movement causing spitting of blood and epistaxis	Cough with spitting of blood, epistaxis or hemoptysis
Guan	Intestine and stomach pain	Qi and blood pain in the lateral costal regions, liver not storing the blood causing spitting of blood and dimming of vision	Intestinal abscess with precipitation of blood, vomiting of blood, no appetite
Chi	Hematuria, red dysentery, uterine bleeding	Lower abdominal precipitation of blood, hemorrhoidal bleeding, women's uterine bleeding	Hemafecia, hematuria, women's menstrual pain

14. *Xian Mai*, Wiry Pulse

	Bin Hu Mai Xue	Left	Right
Cun	Headache, excessive phlegm in the diaphragm	Heart palpitations, headache, night sweats	Chest fullness, phlegmy cough, shortness of breath
Guan	Left: Cold and hot, concretions and conglomerations. Right: Stomach cold	Lateral costal fullness & pain, alternating chills and fever, concretions & conglomerations	Stomach cold, abdominal pain
Chi	Yin *shan*, cramping in both legs	Lower abdominal, lower back & knee aching & pain	Cold *shan*, leg contraction & cramping

15. *Ru Mai,* Soggy Pulse

	Bin Hu Mai Xue	Left	Right
Cun	Yang is slight; spontaneous sweating	Heart vacuity, fright palpitations, chest fullness, shortness of breath, night sweats, loss of sleep	Cough counterflow, fear of cold, chest oppression, shortness of breath, spontaneous perspiration
Guan	Qi vacuity	Lateral costal distention, fullness and discomfort, heart vexation, tendency to get angry, blood not constructing the sinews, sinew contraction, aching & pain	Spleen/stomach vacuity weakness, stomach and epigastric distention & oppression, vacuity swelling, bodily fatigue, torpid intake
Chi	Damaged essence and blood, vacuity cold if severe	Damaged essence in males, blood desertion in females, low back & leg soreness & pain	Vacuity chill of the lower origin, intestinal vacuity diarrhea, loose stools, chilled limbs

16. *Ruo Mai,* Weak Pulse

	Bin Hu Mai Xue	Left	Right
Cun	Yang vacuity diseases	Heart qi vacuity, fright palpitations, spontaneous perspiration, chest fullness, shortness of breath, dizziness, loss of sleep	Qi vacuity, chilled body, chest fullness, shortness of breath
Guan	Stomach weakness and spleen debility	Lateral costal distention, heart vexation, qi depression not soothed, stomach fullness, scanty appetite	Spleen/stomach vacuity weakness, epigastric fullness, abdominal distention, scanty appetite, torpid intake
Chi	Falling of yang, yin vacuity disease	Dizziness, tinnitus, low back soreness, spermatorrhea, kidney origin vacuity, polyuria	Lower abdominal chilly pain, loose stools, devitalized eating and drinking

17. *San Mai*, Scattered Pulse

	Bin Hu Mai Xue	Left	Right
Cun	Left: Fright palpitations. Right: Occasional sweating	Fright palpitations	Sweating
Guan	Left: Spilling over of rheum if soft and scattered. Right: Swollen feet if soft and scattered	Scattered & soft; overflowing rheum	Swollen instep
Chi	Ethereal soul cut off	If both cubit positions are scattered, yin & yang are on the verge of separating	

18. *Xi Mai,* Fine Pulse

	Bin Hu Mai Xue	Left	Right
Cun	Due to frequent vomiting	Racing heart, loss of sleep	Cough counterflow, shortness of breath, chest fullness
Guan	Abdominal distention, stomach vacuity, emaciation	Liver yin vacuity detriment	Spleen vacuity, abdominal oppression
Chi	Chill in the *dan tian*; diarrhea, dysentery, spermatorrhea, yin desertion	Diarrhea, dysentery, spermatorrhea	Lower origin chilly & exhausted

19. *Fu Mai,* Hidden Pulse

	Bin Hu Mai Xue	Left	Right
Cun	Food depression within the chest, desire to vomit but no vomiting	Head dizziness & pain, chest oppression, heart palpitations, shortness of breath	Chest fullness, shortness of breath, cough, rapid breathing, excessive phlegm, hard glomus within the chest
Guan	Abdominal pain causing lethargy	Liver qi surging upward, dizziness, lateral costal distention, heart vexation, tendency to get angry, no thought for food or drink	Stomach & epigastric distention & fullness, no thought for food, accumulation & gathering, aching & pain with the epigastrium
Chi	*Shan* pain as if the abdomen would break	Kidney vacuity, low back pain, lower abdominal distention & fullness, *shan* conglomeration cold pain	Chilly pain below the navel, cold qi contracture and cramping

9
The Pulse in Gynecology

Gynecology is one of the most important and effective specialties in TCM, and the pulse plays as important a part in diagnosis in gynecology as it does in internal medicine. Women differ from men in several regards, not the least of which is the fact that they have a uterus and menstrual cycle and can become pregnant and give birth. Because of these differences, there are some things that practitioners should consider when examining the pulse in women.

The Normal Woman's Pulse

Typically, women's pulses are weaker than men's, slightly deeper and calmer.

The Pulse & Menstruation

Typically, just before the period comes or during the movement of the period, the six pulses will be surging (*hong*), large (*da*), slippery (*hua*), and uninhibited (*li*), or both bar positions may be wiry (*xian*). During the period, these are normal pulses. If there is blood heat in the *chong* and *ren* the pulse will be slippery (*hua*) and rapid (*shu*) or wiry (*xian*) and rapid (*shu*). If yang qi is vacuous and weak and the *chong* and *ren* insufficient, the pulse will be deep (*chen*), slow (*chi*), and fine (*xi*). If there is common cold due to wind cold with the period with evils and blood both slight, the pulse will be floating (*fu*) and tight (*jin*) or floating (*fu*) and slow (*chi*) but with force (*you li*). If there is liver qi depression and binding, qi stagnation and blood stasis, the pulses will be wiry (*xian*), strong (*jing*), and choppy (*se*). If qi and blood are insufficient with the blood chamber empty and vacuous, the pulses will be fine (*xi*) and forceless (*wu li*). If there is excessive discharge of blood with qi and blood both deserting, the pulses will be vacuous (*xu*), large (*da*), and scallion-stalk like (*kong*).

The Pulse & Vaginal Discharge

If vaginal disease pertains to spleen vacuity with exuberant dampness, the pulse will be mostly relaxed (*huan*) and slippery (*hua*). If kidney qi is vacuous and has sustained detriment with abnormal vaginal discharge disease, the foot pulses will mostly be deep (*chen*), weak (*ruo*), and forceless (*wu li*). If vaginal discharge pertains to damp heat smoldering and becoming exuberant, then the pulses mostly will be wiry (*xian*) and rapid (*shu*) or slippery (*hua*) and rapid (*shu*). If cold and dampness have entered and assailed, the pulses will mostly be deep (*chen*) and slow (*chi*).

The Pulse & Pregnancy

During the early part of pregnancy, the pulse will be slippery (*hua*), especially at the inch position. In the late stage of pregnancy, the six pulses may become deep (*chen*), fine (*xi*), short (*duan*), and choppy (*se*) or both cubit positions may be weak (*ruo*). Mostly this is due to kidney qi vacuity weakness or qi and blood dual vacuity. This may also be the case in stirring fetus miscarriage.

The Pulse Postpartum

Postpartum, the qi and blood are vacuous and deficient and the pulses tend to be vacuous (*xu*), relaxed (*huan*), level (*ping*), and harmonious (*he*). Right after delivery, because there is yin and blood vacuity with yang qi exuberant, the pulses may, for a short period of time, be felt to be rapid (*shu*) but in not too long a time, their movement will be felt to be harmonious (*he*) and moderate (*huan*). If postpartum the yin and blood are even more vacuous, vacuous yang may float upward or, postpartum, there may be external invasion of replete evils. In that case, the pulses will be floating (*fu*), slippery (*hua*), and rapid (*shu*). If postpartum there is discharge of blood which will not stop, the pulses may be seen to be fine (*xi*), faint (*wei*), and choppy (*se*). And if there is spontaneous postpartum sweating, one may mainly see a fine (*xi*) and rapid (*shu*) pulse image.

The Main Pulse Images & Their Gynecological Indications

1. ***Fu Mai,* Floating Pulse:** If the pulse is floating, rapid, and forceful at both *cun* positions and if there is no external invasion or exterior pattern, this is categorized as a normal pulse of menstruation. If the pulse is floating and forceless, this is due to qi and blood dual vacuity. This can be seen in flooding and leaking which has endured for days or with a lochia which does not cease.

2. ***Chen Mai,* Deep Pulse:** Water dampness stoppage and retention, qi and blood vacuity weakness, yang qi insufficiency, or qi stagnation and lack of movement, in all these cases one can see a deep pulse. Mostly it is seen after menstruation or in case of blocked menstruation, painful menstruation, swelling and distention during pregnancy, dead fetus which is not precipitated, or agalactia.

3. ***Chi Mai,* Slow Pulse:** This is mostly due to cold exuberance. It can be seen in cases of painful menstruation, blocked menstruation, and infertility.

4. ***Shu Mai,* Rapid Pulse:** Typically, this is mainly associated with heat. If the pulse is rapid and forceful, this is due to repletion. This can be seen in case of early menstruation with excessive amount and flooding and leaking in the initial stage. If the pulse is rapid and forceless, this is due to vacuity. This can be seen in early periods with scanty amount and flooding and leaking in its middle and latter stages.

5. ***Hong Mai,* Surging Pulse:** This is mainly due to heat and yang exuberance. It can be seen in cases of early menstruation with excessive amount, flooding and leaking in its initial stage, and restless fetus precipitating blood.

6. *Hua Mai,* **Slippery Pulse:** If the left *cun* is slippery and uninhibited or both *chi* are slippery and uninhibited and the menses have been stopped and blocked for 2-3 months or more, this is a normal pulse of pregnancy. This also is mainly due to damp exuberance and is mostly seen in vaginal discharge diseases.

7. *Xian Mai,* **Wiry Pulse:** This is mainly due to qi stagnation and is mainly associated with aching and pain. It is mostly seen in case of menstrual irregularity, painful menstruation, blocked menstruation, abdominal pain during pregnancy, postpartum pain and tetany, fetal epilepsy, and concretions and conglomerations.

8. *Jin Mai,* **Tight Pulse:** This is mainly due to coldand is mainly associated with pain. It can be seen in cases of late periods, scanty menstruation or blocked menstruation, painful menstruation, abdominal pain during pregnancy, a lochia which does not move, and postpartum abdominal pain.

9. *Xi Mai,* **Fine Pulse:** This is mainly due to yin vacuity and blood scantiness. It can be seen in case of delayed menstruation, scanty menstruation, and postpartum fever.

10. *Ruo Mai,* **Weak Pulse:** This is mainly due to qi and blood dual vacuity. Mostly it can be seen in cases of delayed menstruation, scanty menstruation or blocked menstruation, dead fetus not being precipitated, and agalactia. It can also be seen in flooding and leaking which has endured for days.

11. *Kou Mai,* **Scallion-stalk Pulse:** This is mainly due to yin and blood sudden collapse. This is mostly seen in case of flooding and leaking precipitation of blood and excessively great loss of blood postpartum.

12. *Se Mai,* **Choppy Pulse:** A choppy pulse without force is due to blood vacuity. A choppy pulse with force is mainly due to blood stasis. It is mostly seen in delayed menstruation with scanty amount, blocked menstruation, infertility, and postpartum blood dizziness.

10
Traditional Pulse Lore Contained in Mnemonic Verse

One of the most difficult things about TCM is that there is so much information which must be memorized if one is going to make this system work. This is one of the reasons that Chinese medicine prizes its *lao yi sheng* or old doctors. It simply takes a long time to learn and assimilate all the facts of TCM to the point where one can think quickly, accurately, and creatively within this system. Therefore, anything which makes the memorization of these facts easier is a boon in mastering this system. Traditionally, most of the basic factual information needed to successfully practice TCM was taught by memorization of mnemonic verses. The information was set to meter and verse, usually arranged in couplets, each line having four, five, or six characters. Students thus sung their lessons, and, just as most readers can still sing their Mother Goose nursery rhymes, these verse couplets had a way of sticking in practitioners' minds throughout their lifelong practice.

Below are translations of a number of such mnemonic verses relating to the pulse. These are taken from the *Zhong Yi Mai Xue Ru Men (Entering the Gate of the Study of the Pulse in Chinese Medicine)*. Actually, the entire *Bin Hu Mai Xue (The Lakeside Master's Study of the Pulse)* is written in verse and its authors intended, nay expected, its students to memorize it. The translations below are not rendered in metered verse. However, they are presented for the information they contain. The more one can read about the pulse and the more one can think about the main pulse images from different perspectives, the more one will remember them. And, if one remembers them, one has the chance of feeling them.

The Various Types of Pulse Images

The pulse has 30 [types]
Which rule the tens of thousands [times] thousands of diseases.

The floating, deep, slow, and fast,
Vacuous, replete, hollow, and wiry,
Surging, minute, long, and short,
Slippery, choppy, tight, and relaxed,
Hidden, fine, drumskin, and confined,
Racing, bound, weak, and soft,
Regularly interrupted pulses [are all] disease pulses.
Besides there is the stirring and scattered.

Pay close attention to each of these abnormal [changes];
Use your heart [*i.e.*, concentration] in studying these intensively.

The Pulse & the Six Environmental Excesses

The six environmental excesses are wind, fire,
Summerheat, dampness, dryness, and cold.

In spring there is wind, in summer, summerheat, and in long summer, dampness pesters.
In winter there is cold, in fall, dryness, and when heat is extreme, fire scorches.

The summerheat pulse is large and rapid; the wind pulse is seen to be wiry.
The fire pulse is surging and rapid; the dryness pulse has two participations.[1]
The cold pulse is slow and tight; and the dampness pulse is somewhat soft.

---

[1] Dryness combines with either damp or cool. Therefore, the pulse will be different depending upon with which of these dryness is combined, heat making the pulse floating and rapid, cool or cold making it floating, tight and slow.

The Pulse & the Seven Affects

If the seven affects damage internally,
They harass and cause chaos to yin and yang.

If the qi dynamic becomes chaotic,
The viscera and bowels lose their normalcy.

If detriment affects the pulse,
The blood's abode is not well.

The spirit and will grind against each other and become chaotic,
And the heart loses its quiet and well-being.

Anger causes the qi to rise,
And blood ejection is difficult to defend against.

Worry and anxiety result in detriment
Affecting the spleen, stomach, and large intestine.

Fear causes the qi to descend
With detriment reaching the kidney viscus.

Sadness leads to scattering of the qi,
And the lung qi suffers disaster.

The Pulse and Static Blood & Phlegm Rheum

If the heart blood becomes static and obstructed,
Chest *bi* will become evident.

If blood stasis occurs in the lungs,
There will be coughing of blood and fishy-smelling phlegm.

If there are concretions and lumps inside the abdomen,
Women will have menstrual pain.

If phlegm turbidity attacks the heart,
There will be mania, *bi*, and palpitations.

If phlegm rheum damages the lungs,
There will be cough and wheezing with the sound of phlegm.

If there is phlegm inside the channels and connecting vessels,
There will be wind stroke with crying out involuntarily.
Phlegm and rheum engender hundreds of diseases crowding together.

The blood stasis pulse is choppy,
And the pulse corresponding to phlegm is slippery.

The Song of Eight Principles Pattern Discrimination, Pulse & Tongue, Patterns & Treatment

If the pulse is floating, the disease is in the exterior,
While if the pulse is deep, this pertains to an interior pattern.

A slow pulse pertains to cold for sure and one can lean on this,
While one should remember that a rapid pulse is associated with heat patterns.

In vacuity patterns, [the pulse is] vacuous, fine, soft, weak, and small,
While in repletion patterns, the pulse is replete and torrential.

The pulse of exterior cold is floating and tight,
While a floating and relaxed [pulse] is an exterior vacuity [for which] secure the skin and hair.

A floating and rapid pulse is exterior heat which can be harmonized at daybreak,
While a floating, tight pulse is exterior repletion which should be treated by the sweating method.

A deep, slow [pulse] is interior cold, for which warming and scattering are good.
A deep, rapid [pulse] is interior heat which can be dissipated by cooling medicinals.

An interior vacuity's pulse is weak and it is appropriate to treat it early.
An interior repletion has a replete, deep pulse; look in the center.

For vacuity patterns of the four kinds, it is appropriate to supplement with medicinals.
But, yin and yang, qi and blood, do not mix these up.

In yin vacuity, [the pulse is] fine and rapid and fluids and blood are scant.
In yang vacuity, the pulse is weak; warm and supplement with expensive [ingredients].

In qi vacuity, the pulse is vacuous, [for which] Four Gentlemen are miraculous.
In blood vacuity, the pulse is fine, [which] Four Materials regulates.

In yin collapse and yang collapse, [either] fluids or qi may be consumed.
The pulse and pattern combined must be finely considered.

In yin collapse, a fine, rapid, and soft pulse is the omen,
While in yang collapse, the pulse is minute, weak, and on the verge of withering.

The Song of Qi & Blood Pattern Discrimination, Pulse & Tongue, Patterns & Treatment

Qi and blood pulses and patterns are several times seven;
The treatment methods of these pulses and patterns are not the same.

With qi vacuity there is shortness of breath, fatigue, and lack of strength,
Vertigo, dizziness, a pale tongue, and a vacuous pulse.

With qi fall, urination is numerous and there is abdominal sagging and glomus;
If the pulse is vacuous and desertion is severe, this is mostly due to fatigue.

With qi stagnation, there is aching and pain, glomus, oppression and *bi*;
If the pulse is mostly slippery and replete, regulate the qi mechanism.

With qi counterflow, there is cough, panting, vomiting, and hiccup,
Headache, dizziness, inversion, and a wiry, slippery sign.

With blood vacuity, there is lack of luster and excessive fright palpitations;
Thus there is seen bleeding, pain, swelling, and stasis.

With blood heat, the pulse is rapid and the tongue is scarlet;
There is bleeding, dimness, mania, vexation, agitation, and urgency.

11
The Rhymed Formula of the Heart Methods of the Pulse

The following is a translation of the 34th *juan* of the *Yi Zong Jin Jian (Golden Mirror of Ancestral Medicine)*. Published in 1742 CE, this 90 *juan* medical encyclopedia was compiled by a staff of 80 doctors under the famous court physician Wu Qian. This encyclopedia codified most of what was valuable and effective in Chinese medicine up to that time and is one of the main premodern sources of what has now come to be known as TCM. The 34th *juan* of the *Yi Zong Jin Jian* is titled "The Rhymed Formula of the Essential Heart Methods of the Four Examinations." It is divided into upper or first and lower or second chapters. The second chapter has to do with pulse examination. As with so many other topics, modern TCM pulse examination is largely based on this compendium. Therefore, I have chosen to translate its section on the pulse in its entirety.

The vessels [a.k.a. the pulse] are the mansion of the blood.
They penetrate and flow freely through the hundreds [of parts of] the body.
The stirring [*i.e.*, pulsing] vessel at the *cun kou*
Is their great reunion, the courtyard of their master.

The examination of the pulse
Should be taken on top of the high bone.
Therefore it is called the bar
Because it separates the inch and cubit.

From the fish's [belly, *i.e.*, the thenar eminence] is one inch.

From the pool [*i.e.*, *Chi Ze* {Lu 5}] is one cubit.
Therefore they are assigned these names.
The inch is yang and the foot is yin.

The right inch [corresponds to] the lungs and chest,
The left inch to the heart and center of the chest,
The right bar to the spleen and stomach,
The left to the liver, diaphragm, and gallbladder.

The three sections [correspond to] the three burners.
Both cubits [correspond to] the two kidneys,
The left [also] to the small [intestine and] bladder,
And the right [also] to the large intestine.

The life gate pertains to the kidneys.
It is the source of living qi.
If the two cubits are absent in a person,
There must be death and no recovery.

The bar pulse [measures] one inch.
The right [corresponds to] food and the left to wind.
The right is the *qi kou* [qi mouth],
And the left is the *ren ying* [human prognosis].

The pulse has seven [places of] examination.
Floating, middle, and deep,
Upper [*i.e.*, distal] and lower [*i.e.*, proximal],
Left and right [should these] be pushed and searched.

A man's left should be normally large,
While a woman's right is appropriately large.
A man's cubit is usually vacuous,
While a woman's cubit is usually replete.

There are also [another] three sections.

These are called heaven, earth, and human.
Since each section has three [divisions],
Thus there are nine places of which to inquire.

[Heaven section pulses are found at] the forehead, cheeks, and in front of the ears.
[Earth section pulses are found at] the inch opening, the thumb-forefinger joint, and styloid process.
[Human section pulses are found at] the three yin on the lower foot,
The liver, kidney, and spleen/stomach.[1]

At the great reunion of the inch opening,
[If the pulse stops once in] fifty [beats], this is consistent with the channels [*i.e.*, normal].
[If it stops in] less than [that number of] beats,
There is no qi and [this is] necessarily ominous.

If, in addition, it is coursing and rapid,
Stops, but is unable [to make up this pause],
Shortly there will be death within one year.
This is fixed and it is difficult for one to live.

The five viscera have their root pulses
And each of these have their norms.
The heart [pulse] is floating, large, and scattered.
The lung [pulse] is floating, choppy, and short.

---

[1] This stanza refers to taking the pulse at the following nine sites: *Tai Yang* (M-HN-9), *Er Men* (TH 21), *Jia Che* (St 36), *Tai Yuan* (Lu 9), *Shen Men* (Ht 7), *He Gu* (LI 4), *Wu Li* (Liv 10), *Jin Men* (Sp 11), *Tai Xi* (Ki 3).

The liver [pulse] is deep, wiry, and long.
The kidney [pulse] is deep, slippery, and soft.
In any case, it should be tolerant [*i.e.*, peaceful, full, and uninhibited] and harmonious.
The spleen center is slow and relaxed.

The level [*i.e.*, normal] pulse of the four seasons
Should be relaxed, harmonious, and even.
In spring, wiry, and in summer, surging;
In fall, hair-like, and in winter, deep.

When the pulse is too replete and strong,
Disease is engendered in the outside.
If it does not reach and is vacuous and faint,
Disease is engendered in the inside.

If drinking and eating [are undisciplined] and there is overtaxation and fatigue,
Examine the right and left bars.
If they have force, this is repletion,
While if they are forceless, this is vacuity.

When examining the disease pulse,
[Doing it at] dawn is the most accurate.
[The physician should be] empty and still with a calm heart,
Regulated respiration, and a fine and careful trial.

One inhalation, one exhalation,
Together they make one respiration.
If the pulse comes four [times to one respiration],
Moderate is normal.

If it comes five [times] this is not diseased
Because of the interval between a great respiration.
Three times is slow,
And slow means there is chill.

Six times is fast,
And fast means there is a hot pattern.
If moderately slow, there is moderate chill;
If moderately fast, there is moderate heat.

Once slow and fast are clear,
Then floating and deep forms must be distinguished.
Floating, deep, slow, and fast,
These discriminate internal and external causes.

External causes come from heaven.
Internal causes come from humans.
Heaven has yin and yang,
Wind, rain, darkness, and brightness.
In humans, there are joy, worry, anger,
Thinking, sorrow, fear, and fright.

Once floating and deep have been discriminated,
Slippery and choppy should be made clear.
Choppy is due to blood stasis;
Slippery is due to qi congestion.

A floating pulse is a skin pulse [*i.e.*, it can be felt at the level of the skin].
A deep pulse [is felt at the level of] the sinews and bone.
At the muscles and flesh is found the middle [level].
Thus each section's place is subordinated.

Floating without force is soggy.
Deep without force is weak.
Deep and extremely forceful is confined.
Floating and extremely forceful is drumskin.

If the three sections have force,
This is also called replete.
If the three sections lack force,
This is also called vacuous.

If the three sections are forceless,
If when pressing it is small,
Sometimes it is there and sometimes not,
A faint pulse can be verified.

If the three sections are forceless,
If when pressing it is large,
If it vanishes and floods and is unable to collect itself together,
A scattered pulse can be scrutinized.

If only the middle is forceless,
This is also called scallion-stalk.
[If only felt when] pushing the sinews and touching the bone,
The hidden pulse can be seen.

If three [beats] arrive [per respiration], this is slow;
If six arrive, this is fast.
If four arrive, this is relaxed;
If seven arrive, this is a racing pulse.

If relaxed and stops, this is called bound;
If rapid and stops, this is called skipping [or rapid irregularly interrupted pulse].
In examining both of these,
They are each connected and arrive with their number [*i.e.*, they make up for the loss].

If [the pulse] beats and stops in the middle
And is not able to recuperate itself,
They arrive but their number is not correct [*i.e.*, they are not able to make up for the loss],
[Such] a regularly interrupted [pulse] means a difficult recovery.

Shaped like a pearl,
The slippery [pulse] is flowing and unstable.
If it comes astringent and stagnant,
This is evidence of a choppy pulse.

If wiry, fine, and straight,
All these characteristics are called wiry.
A tight [pulse] is thicker than a wiry [pulse].
Its expression is that it is elastic to the left and right.

If it comes exuberantly but departs debilitatedly,
This is called a surging pulse.
A large [pulse] means that it is wide.
A small [pulse] means it is fine and diminished [*i.e.*, narrow].

[A stirring pulse] is like a bean chaotically stirring.
It shakes without moving [its place].
[A pulse which travels] far and far is long,
[While a pulse which is] drawn back and contracted is short.

A floating, yang [pulse] is mainly an exterior [condition],
Wind and the six environmental excess qi.
If it has force, this is an exterior repletion;
If it is forceless, this is an exterior vacuity.

If floating and slow, this is an exterior chill;
If floating and relaxed, this is wind dampness.
If floating and soggy, this is damage due to summerheat.
If floating and scattered, this is extreme vacuity.

If floating and surging, this is yang exuberance;
If floating and large, this is yang repletion.
If floating and fine, this is scanty qi;
If floating and choppy, this is blood vacuity.

If floating and rapid, this is wind heat;
If floating and tight, this is wind cold.
If floating and wiry, this is wind rheum;
If floating and slippery, this is wind phlegm.

A deep, yin [pulse] is mainly an interior [condition],
The seven affects, qi, and food.
If deep and large, this is interior repletion;
If deep and small, this is interior vacuity.

If deep and slow, this is interior chill.
If deep and relaxed, this is interior dampness.
If deep and tight, this is chilly pain.
If deep and rapid, this is interior heat.

If deep and choppy, this is interior *bi* qi.
If deep and slippery, this is phlegm food.
If deep and hidden, this is blockage and depression.
If deep and wiry, this is a rheum disease.

A soggy [pulse] is a yang vacuity disease,
While a wiry [pulse] is a yin vacuity disease.
A faint [pulse] rules all vacuities.
[If the pulse is] scattered, vacuity is severe.

A drumskin [pulse] is damage to essence blood,
Half delivery [*i.e.*, miscarriage], *dai* [*xia*], or *beng*.
A confined [pulse] is *shan*, concretion and conglomerations,
Heart and abdominal cold pain.

A vacuous [pulse] rules all kinds of vacuity;
A replete [pulse] rules all kinds of repletions.
A scallion-stalk [pulse] is mainly loss of blood.
Following what is seen, one can know [what the condition is].

A slow [pulse means] cold mainly in the viscera.
Thus yin [*i.e.*, a visceral condition] and cold are mutually implicated.
If forceful, there is cold pain;
If forceless, vacuity cold.

A rapid [pulse means] heat mainly in the viscera.
If rapid and fine, yin is damaged.
If it has force, this is replete heat.
If it is forceless, this is vacuity sore.

A relaxed [pulse means] dampness of the spleen and stomach.
If [also] tight and large, this is damp congestion.
A skipping [pulse] is yang depression.
A bound [pulse] means yin congelation.

A regularly interrupted [pulse] means qi fatigue,
Fall and strike, oppression, and exhaustion,
Qi retrenchment, painful sores,
And a woman with fetus in the third month.

A slippery [pulse] commands phlegm diseases,
[But at] the bar is mainly food and wind.
At the inch, one can check for vomiting and counterflow.
At the cubit, there may be bloody, pussy stools.

A choppy [pulse means] vacuity, dampness, or *bi*.
In the cubit, [it means] essence blood damage;
In the inch, sweating of fluids and thirst;
In the bar, lower esophageal obstruction and perishing of fluids.

A wiry [pulse in the] bar is mainly rheum
Or wood insulting the spleen channel.
If the inch is wiry, [this means] headache.
If the cubit is wiry, [this means] abdominal pain.

A tight [pulse] mainly [means] cold pain.
A surging [pulse] is fire damage.
A stirring [pulse] mainly [means] pain and heat,
Beng, sweating, fright, and mania.

A long [pulse] means qi is in order,
While a short [pulse] means qi is diseased.
A fine [pulse] means qi is debilitated,
While a big [pulse] means the disease is advancing.

The pulse *vis à vis* the main disease
May be appropriate and may be inappropriate.
Yin and yang, normal flow and counterflow,
Auspicious or ill-omened, one can infer.

The pulse of wind stroke
Should be floating and slow.
If it is tight and large, urgent and racing,
This is ominous and one can know [the prognosis].

In damage by cold or heat disease,
The pulse should be floating and surging.
If deep, faint, choppy, or small,
This is contrary to the pattern and is necessarily ominous.

After sweating, if the pulse is still
And the body is cool, this leads to quiet.
After sweating, if the pulse is agitated
And fever is severe, this must be difficult [to cure].

If a yang pattern manifests yin [pulses],
One's destiny must necessarily be in great danger.
If a yin pattern manifests yang [pulses],
Although [one may be] hard-pressed, [there will be] no calamity.

If taxation and fatigue damage the spleen,
The pulse should be vacuous and weak,
[But if there is] spontaneous sweating and an agitated pulse,
Death cannot be driven back.

If there is inhibited diarrhea,
[The pulse should be] deep, small, slippery, and weak.
If replete, large, floating, and rapid
With fever, this means a malign [condition].

If there is vomiting and stomach reflux,
And [the pulse] is floating, slippery, this is auspicious.
If deep, rapid, fine, and choppy,
Then the colon is [affected and there will be] perishing.

In terms of cholera-like disease,
If the pulse is regularly interrupted, no surprise.
But if the tongue is curled and the testes shrunken,
[There is cold] hidden in the *jue* [*yin*] and this can be [cause for] lament.

In cough, the pulse [should be] mostly floating.
If floating and soggy, an easy cure.
If deep, hidden, and tight,
Death is about to arrive.

If there is dyspnea and lifting the shoulders with breathing
And [the pulse is] floating and slippery, this is normal.
If deep and choppy with cold limbs,
This is an inauspicious pattern.

In diseases of fire and heat,
Surging, rapid [pulses] are appropriate.
If faint and weak, [there is] no spirit;
It has deserted and separated from the root.

In steaming bone fever,
The pulse [should be] rapid and vacuous.
If there is fever and [the pulse] is choppy and small,
The body must die.

[In case of] extreme taxation and all kinds of vacuity,
[The pulse should be] floating, soft, faint, and weak.
But if both [bars] are wiry, then earth is vanquished,
And if fine and rapid, there is fire flaring.

In all patterns of blood loss,
The pulse must appear scallion-stalk.
If relaxed and small, one can be joyous,
But if rapid and large, this is critical.

If there is retention of blood in the center,
A confined, large pulse is appropriate.
If deep, choppy, and faint,
A rapid recovery is rare.

If the pulse of the three dispersions [*i.e.*, diabetes]
Is rapid and large, all live.
If fine, faint, short, and choppy,
The responding hand [*i.e.*, the physician] should feel fright.

If there is urinary strangury and blockage,
The color of the nose must be yellow.
If there is a replete, large [pulse], it can be treated,
But if choppy and small, know [that the patient will] perish.

If withdrawal reaches double yin
And mania reaches double yang,
A floating, surging [pulse] is a good sign.
Deep and urgent, it is inauspicious and brings disaster.

In epilepsy [the pulse] should be floating and relaxed.
If deep, small, urgent, and replete, [it means the disease is deep].
If it is wiry and without stomach,
[The patient] must inevitably die.

Heart and abdominal pain,
There are nine types of this.
If fine and slow, there may be a speedy cure.
If floating, and large, [the disease] will be long enduring.

Shan is categorized as a liver disease;
Therefore, its pulse must be wiry and tense.
If it is confined and tense, all will live.
If it is weak and tense, all will die.

In damp heat jaundice,
If [the pulse] is surging and rapid, this is appropriate.
[It is also] not alarming if it is floating and large.
If faint and choppy, this is a difficult disease.

The pulse of swelling and distention [*i.e.*, edema]
Should be floating, large, surging, and replete.
If fine, deep, and faint,
Qi [Bo and] Huang [Di] have no art [which can cure it].

[In case of] accumulations in the five viscera
And gatherings in the six bowels,
If [the pulse] is replete and strong, one can live,
But if deep and fine, they are difficult to cure.

[In case of] nausea and abdominal distention,
If [the pulse] is tight and fine, there will be life.
If floating and large, what?
Evil qi is already flourishing.

The pulse of ghost possession
Is not even on the right and left.
Suddenly it is large and suddenly small;
Suddenly it is rapid and suddenly it is slow.

In *yong* and *ju* without eruption,
The pulse should be surging and large.
If it has already ruptured,
A surging large [pulse] is contraindicated.

If a lung abscess has already formed,
The inch should be rapid and replete.
In the pattern of lung consumption,
[The pulse] is rapid and forceless.

In abscess and consumption with white-colored [face],
The pulse should be short and choppy.
If one meets a rapid and large [pulse],
Qi has suffered detriment and blood has been lost.

In intestinal abscess due to replete heat,
Slippery, rapid [pulses] are mutually appropriate [to the disease].
If deep, fine, and without root,
Death can occur in one year.

When a woman is with child,
The yin [pulse] beat and the yang will be different.
If the *shao yin* beats strongly,
The fetus is already bound.

If slippery, racing, and scattered,
The fetus must be in the third month.
If pressure does not scatter it,
It can be known to be in the fifth month.

[If slippery] on the left, a boy, on the right, a girl.
During pregnancy, there may be lactation.
If a girl, the abdomen will be like a winnowing basket.
If a boy, the abdomen will be like a cauldron.

Immediately prior to delivery, [the pulse] may depart from the norm.
In the newly delivered, [the pulse should be] small and relaxed.
If replete, wiry, confined, and large,
A bad omen cannot be dismissed.

Normal pulses and disease pulses
Have already been described in detail.
Next will be handled [those dealing with] the expiry of the body
With the same sort of measure and weight [*i.e.*, detail].

The pulse of heart expiry
Is like grasping a hook on a belt.
[If it appears] agitated and racing like a spinning bean,
In one day one can die.

The pulse of liver expiry
Is like touching the blade of a knife.
[If it appears] wiry like a newly strung bow,
Death will be in eight days.

The spleen expiry [pulse] is like a sparrow pecking.
It may also be like a roof leaking.
In addition, it may be like pouring water from a cup.
No rescue on the fourth day.

What is the dimension [of the pulse] of lung expiry?
It is like wind blowing through the hair
Or a feather striking the skin.
Three days and wailing.

What is [the pulse] of kidney expiry?
It is emitted like a taught cord
Or like tapping one's fingers on a stone.
In four days it will happen.

The life [gate] pulse when it expires
Is like a fish hovering or shrimp swimming.
It may also arrive like a bubbling spring.
Nothing can persuade [the patient] to stay.

There is also the pulse on the back of the wrist
Which beats on the back of the arm,
Stemming from *Lie Que* [*i.e.*, Lu 7].
This has nothing to do with the knowing of patterns.

Qi [Bo and] Huang [Di developed] pulse technique
[In order to] examine diseases [and distinguish] death from life.
[Later, in terms of] the *Tai Su* pulse technique,[2]
[There are both] yin and yang noble, clear [pulses].

Clear [pulses] are like moist jade;
They arrive with their numerous [beats] clearly divided.
Turbid [pulses] are like stone;
Their appearance is like plaster [*i.e.*, dull and] not clear.

Small and large [equal] impoverished or wealthy.
Choppy and slippery [equal] poverty-stricken or free flowing.
Long and short [equal] long life or young death.
[Thus] detailed inferences [can be made about] complex [situations].

---

2 This refers to the Ming Dynasty book *Tai Su Mai Mi Jue (Tai Su's Secret Rhymes of the Pulse)* by Zhang Tai-su.

12
Unusual Pulse Images

In TCM, there are 10 pulse images above and beyond the main 27-29 that all have to do with extremely critical conditions. These are called the *shi guai mai*, the ten strange pulses. These are not commonly encountered in the out-patient clinic. I do not know that I have ever felt them. They are presented here merely for the sake of completeness. The reader should note, however, that these are not some completely other pulse images. Rather, they are only extreme forms of the main pulse images described and discussed above. Therefore, I do not think these 10 pulse images need to be memorized. Their extreme qualities should alert every practitioner to the seriousness of their indications in any case.

1. ***Que Zhuo Mai,* Pecking Pulse:** This pulse is urgent and rapid, its discipline and restraint are irregular, and it sometimes stops and then begins again. It is likened to a sparrow pecking while feeding and thus its name.

2. ***Wu Lou Mai,* Leaking Roof Pulse:** This pulse is extremely slow and arrhythmic. Its pulses are, therefore, likened to water dripping through a leaky roof, one beat every now and then.

3. ***Tan Shi Mai,* Flicking Pulse:** This pulse is deep and replete. It feels like a finger tapping on stone, it is so hard and tight.

4. ***Jie Suo Mai,* Untying Rope Pulse:** This pulse suddenly flows and suddenly stops. Therefore, it is extremely irregular in rhythm and frequency.

5. *Yu Xiang Mai,* **Waving Fish Pulse:** This pulse is barely palpable as if it almost were not there.

6. *Xia You Mai,* **Darting Shrimp Pulse:** This pulse is sometimes very indistinct and faint and sometimes distinct.

7. *Fu Fei Mai,* **Seething Cauldron Pulse:** This pulse is extremely floating and rapid. It is, therefore, like the bubbles of boiling water.

8. *Yan Dao Mai,* **Upturned Knife Pulse:** This pulse iswiry and fine, tight and tense. It is like feeling the edge of a knife.

9. *Zhuan Dou Mai,* **Spinning Bean Pulse:** This pulse comes unpredictably and without stability. Therefore, it is traditionally likened to being as hard to catch as peas rolling around a dish.

10. *Ma Cu Mai,* **Frenzied Sesame Seed Pulse:** This pulse is extremely rapid and completely chaotic.

13
Reading the Cubit Positions

In terms of reading the meaning of the *cun kou* pulse, there is wide agreement, both historically in Asia and contemporaneously in the West, over the correspondences of the inch and bar positions. However, when it comes to the cubit positions, there is much disagreement and confusion. In the *Nan Jing (Classic of Difficulties)* and the *Mai Jing (Pulse Classic)*, the left cubit corresponds to the hand *shao yang*, *i.e.*, triple burner, superficially and to the hand *jue yin*, *i.e.*, the pericardium, deep, while the right cubit is said to correspond to the foot *tai yang*, bladder, superficially and the foot *shao yin*, kidneys, deep. By the late Ming dynasty with the *Bin Hu Mai Xue (The Lakeside Master's Study of the Pulse)* and the *Jing Yue Quan Shu ([Zhang] Jing-yue's Complete Writings)* and into the Qing with the *Yi Zong Jin Jian (Golden Mirror of Ancestral Medicine)*, most Chinese doctors agreed that the *chi* or cubit positions reflected all the contents of the lower burner and only especially the kidneys. However, Li Shi-zhen and the authors of the *Yi Zong Jin Jian* say that the left cubit corresponds to the kidney, small intestine, and bladder, while Zhang Jing-yue says that the left cubit corresponds to the kidney, bladder, and large intestine. Conversely, Li Shi-zhen believed that the right cubit reflected the life gate and large intestine, while Zhang Jing-yue stated that the right cubit corresponds to the kidney, triple burner, life gate, and small intestine.

Immediately, the seeming discrepancy between the *Nan Jing/Mai Jing* and the *Bin Hu Mai Xue/Yi Zong Jin Jian* regarding the pericardium can be easily explained by quoting Li Dong-yuan:

> Ministerial fire is the fire of the pericardium developing from the lower burner.[1]

Ministerial fire is the life gate fire or kidney fire as opposed to the sovereign fire residing in the heart. As Li correctly states, the fire of the pericardium develops or has its source in the lower burner. Thus one can know something about the pericardium by knowing about the contents of the lower burner. However, it is not so easy to explain why some Chinese authors say the life gate or kidney fire can be read in both cubits, others in the right cubit, or yet others in the left cubit. Nor is it so easy to explain why some authors place the small intestine in the right cubit and large intestine in the left and others place them just the opposite. It is my opinion that the function of the kidneys one places in the right or left cubits and which bowels one places in the right or left cubits has to do with the author's theoretical beliefs about the relationship of kidney water and kidney fire to both the viscera and the bowels.

For years now I have read kidney fire or the life gate fire on the right. This is because of kidney fire's being the source for the transformation of qi and transportation of water which is carried out by the lungs and spleen and which are also read on the right. Because I believe that the source of kidney yang is found in the large intestine, I tend to read the large intestine also in the right cubit. Conversely, I read kidney yin in the left cubit. This is because kidney yin is related to both liver and heart blood. Further, I read the small intestine in the left cubit because of the relationship between the small intestine and kidney yin. I believe my reading of the left and right cubit positions is corroborated by Zhang Wei-yan, a practitioner in Taiwan, who says that the right cubit corresponds to the former heaven (*xian tian*), the triple burner and its fluid metabolism, and the life gate, while the left cubit reflects the latter heaven (*hou tian*), the essence, and the urinary excretion system.

---

1 Li Dong-yuan, *Li Dong-yuan's Treatise on the Spleen & Stomach*, trans. by Yang Shou-zhong & Li Jian-yong, Blue Poppy Press, Boulder, CO, 1993, p. 84

Nonetheless, when reading the cubit pulses, I believe that one must not be doctrinaire but remain flexible and open-minded. Open-minded to what? To the other corroborating signs and symptoms relating to the pelvic contents and to the entire body below the waist. Thus a tight or wiry pulse may not have anything to do with the kidneys or the bowels. Instead, it may be a manifestation of sacroiliac or sciatic pain. Further, it is my experience that the interpretation of the pulse images in the cubit positions should not be read in isolation, but should be read in relationship to the images presented in the other two positions on both hands. For instance, a hooked pulse appears most obviously abnormal in the inch or *cun* position but nevertheless tells one about the failure of the kidneys to root yang in its lower origin.

Abnormal Pulse Images in the Cubit Position

Because the kidneys are the water viscus, their pulse should be somewhat deep, slippery, and have force, but not be wiry or tight. That is the quality of a normal pulse in the *chi* or cubit position. The following pulse images are all abnormal ones when found in the cubit.

Zhang Wei-yan describes six abnormal pulse images in the cubit positions which I think are useful in clarifying the indications of the images found in the cubit position. Zhang's first is a floating and fine left cubit. The floating image suggests yang qi moving upward and outward. Fine suggests a vacuity of yin, blood, and essence. Therefore, this image indicates yin vacuity with yang counterflowing upward. This image is often seen in cases of hormonal imbalance in women, infertility, and menopausal syndrome.

Zhang's second image is a left cubit pulse which is deep, fine, and forceless. This is indicative of yang vacuity with yin exuberance. Yin exuberance here means dampness and cold. The cold is vacuity cold. This pulse image is often seen in cases of enduring illness where kidney yang has been damaged.

Zhang's third abnormal cubit pulse is a deep, wiry, long, large, and forceful right cubit. Dr. Zhang says this indicates damp heat in the lower burner.

This image often corresponds to urinary tract infection with frequent, urgent urination and yellowish red or turbid urine.

Zhang's fourth abnormal cubit pulse is if either the left or right cubit is short, stirring, and forceful. Short means that there is blockage and inhibited flow, while a stirring pulse is often associated with pain. Therefore, this is a common pulse image in cases of urinary tract stones. If the stone is lodged on the right, then this image typically appears on the right, and if the stone is located on the left, this image will appear on the left.

Zhang's fifth abnormal cubit pulse is a left cubit which is deep, wiry, thin, long, and hard like a needle. It has force. This pulse is indicative of a liver blood insufficiency. In that case, liver blood is failing to nourish the sinews and bones. Diseases manifesting this pulse image include various bone diseases, such as osteoporosis and vertebral hyperplasia, and chronic *bi zheng* of different kinds.

Zhang's sixth abnormal cubit pulse image is when the left cubit is deep, scattered, and forceless and the bar and cubit do not connect freely. Dr. Zhang reads this as blood stasis and damp heat. This is sometimes referred to in the Chinese literature simply as stasis heat. It is a common condition among women with endometriosis.

Personally, I have found these pulse images of Dr. Zhang's to be quite accurate. I would also like to add, however, that often one finds a slightly deep, slippery, wiry, forceful pulse in the right cubit at the same time that the left cubit is fine and relatively forceless. In my experience, this commonly found pulse image is seen in cases of damp heat affecting the large intestine which then damages kidney yang. Because of this, ministerial fire tends to counterflow upward, and hence the inch or *cun* positions tend to be floating and rootless or hooked. However, because of the interrelationship between yin and yang and the fact that the spleen is the source of dampness as well as the origin of the engenderment of blood, this condition is often complicated by elements of spleen qi vacuity and dampness as well as blood and yin vacuity. I discuss this pattern further under the heading of yin fire in the following chapter.

14
Yin Fire & the Pulse

Close to twenty years ago when I was first studying Chinese medicine, I felt an old man's pulse. He had water swelling so bad in his lower extremities that, when I acupunctured his legs, water dripped out of the insertion sites after the needles were removed. This man had a large, slippery, somewhat rapid pulse. At the time, I was perplexed. I figured he should have a rapid, fine, and wiry pulse. Nonetheless, I took his pulse images to indicate repletion. When he asked me what I thought of his pulses, I told him that, although he was old and should have fine, weak pulses, he seemed to be very robust and, based on his pulses, he should live a long life. He died less than a year later of cardiopulmonary disease.

The reason I am telling this story is that it is easy to misread the pulse if one does not think deeply about the mechanisms involved in the production of the pulse images. At the time, I was not sensitive to checking to see if pulses were well rooted and not floating. I do not know if this man's pulse was slippery, large, *floating*, and rapid, but in retrospect I think they probably were. If they were, this is a surging pulse. A surging pulse is due to heat, but not necessarily replete heat. Because I did not know the definitions of all the main pulse images, I failed to define this patient's pulse as a surging pulse. Further, I did not understand at the time the mechanisms at work making the pulse images manifest as they do. Therefore, I misread a vacuity pulse for a repletion pulse.

In my experience as a teacher, I find that this is a common mistake. Chinese textbooks and their English language translations always give the fine and rapid pulse as the standard yin vacuity pulse. They also give the deep and slow pulse as the standard yang vacuity pulse. However, it is my experience that most of my patient population suffering from one or even both of these patterns do not exhibit these textbook images. When the pattern is a replete one, I believe the pulse images are, for the most part, pretty straightforward and conform to one's textbook expectations. But when it comes to chronic vacuity conditions and mixed repletion and vacuity patterns, more often than not in my experience, the pulses are something other than the textbook norm. This discrepancy confuses many Western practitioners who then call into question the entire system of TCM, wondering whether TCM patterns actually do fit our Western patients.

It is my experience that TCM patterns do fit our Western patients but not like a ready-made dress taken directly from the rack. Rather, because of the complex and deep-seated reasons discussed in the Introduction for Western patients developing the sorts of difficult, knotty diseases they come to practitioners of acupuncture and TCM to treat, many, and maybe even most, Western patients have complex TCM pattern discriminations. This means that there are a welter of signs and symptoms which frequently look confusing at best and contradictory at worst. This further means that our patients' TCM pattern discriminations must usually be custom-tailored out of pieces or aspects of 2, 3, 4, or even 5 disease mechanisms.

Yin Fire

As mentioned above, I think this problem of complex pattern diagnoses and, therefore, complex pulse images primarily shows up in vacuity or mixed repletion/vacuity conditions. When it comes to chronic, difficult to treat, what the Chinese call knotty diseases, the theory that I have found most helpful to me in my practice has been Li Dong-yuan and Zhu Dan-xi's theory of yin fire and all its ramifications. It is this theory which, I believe, makes sense of a passage such as the following from Hua Tuo's *Zhong Zang Jing (Classic of the Central Viscera)*:

> Kidney disease may be accompanied by counterflow frigidity of the hands and feet, a red facial complexion with yellow eyes, incontinence of urine, tormenting pain of the joints of the bones, binding pain in the lower abdomen, and qi surging upward into the heart. If the pulse is floating, large, and relaxed rather than deep, fine, and slippery as it ought to be and, if the complexion which ought to be black is now otherwise [yellow

> in a variant edition], this is earth coming to conquer water, a greatly adverse [condition].[1]

In this case, already defined by Hua Tuo as a kidney disease, there is at least one unquestionable symptom of kidney yang vacuity: the counterflow frigidity. In the case of kidney yang vacuity, the face should be black or dark and dull and the pulse should be deep and fine. However, the face is red with yellow eyes and the pulse is floating. Hua Tuo says that this is a greatly adverse condition and that it is due to the spleen coming to conquer water. Thus the kidneys become weak and vacuous but qi surges upward tingeing the face red. Yellow is the color associated with the earth spleen and the spleen is associated with dampness. Likewise the relaxed pulse is associated with vacuity and damp conditions. Thus, when Hua Tuo says this is the spleen coming to conquer water, he means that there is dampness damaging the kidneys due to spleen vacuity. It is this which then causes the upward surging of the qi. It is not entirely clear if the tormenting pain in the joints is due to kidney vacuity or that plus a combination of cold dampness or damp heat. Although the mechanism for the binding pain in the lower abdomen is also not explicitly stated, it seems to me we are talking about a combination of dampness and cold or dampness and heat combined with vacuity cold and blood stasis/qi stagnation. Further, Hua Tuo says that in kidney disease one expects to see certain textbook symptoms but, in fact, because the pattern is complicated, one sees quite different ones.

Approximately eleven centuries later, Li Dong-yuan, in his monumental *Pi Wei Lun (Treatise on the Spleen & Stomach)*, further elucidated the mechanisms at work in the above scenario described in the late Han Dynasty by Hua Tuo. Li called such upsurging, counterflowing heat "yin fire". This term yin fire should not be confused with vacuity heat. Although it does share one common mechanism, it is a broader, more complicated, and more inclusive concept. The yin in Li Dong-yuan's yin fire stands for yin cold and dampness generated mostly by a damaged spleen. Due to overthinking and worry, overtaxation, overeating, undereating, and eating the wrong foods, the spleen fails to control transportation and

---

[1] Hua Tuo, *op. cit.*, p 96-97

transformation. The turbid portion of foods and liquids is not separated from the clear and this becomes damp turbidity. This damp turbidity, because it is yin, percolates down into the lower burner, there to damage the liver and kidneys. Because the host qi of the body is yang, damp turbidity often transforms into damp heat. Because of dampness damaging kidney yang and because the heat of damp heat tends to float upward, yang loses its root in its lower source and also tends to surge upward. Thus, although there are symptoms of cold (and possibly damp heat below), there are symptoms of heat above, with other symptoms manifesting vacuity weakness of the spleen.

According to Li Dong-yuan, there are five disease mechanisms which can cause or contribute to yin fire. the first is spleen qi vacuity. The second is damp heat. The third is blood vacuity (*i.e.*, yin vacuity). The fourth is liver depression (*i.e.*, liver invading the spleen and depressive heat). The fifth is stirring of ministerial fire due to extremes of the five or seven affects. For instance:

> Since the spleen and stomach are vacuous, unable to rise or float, their engendering and perfusing qi are damaged by yin fire, *ying* and blood are greatly depleted, and constructive qi is confined to earth. If yin fire burns effulgently, boiling day after day, blood and qi become (more and more) depleted and scant. What's more, because blood is governed by the pericardium and heart, reduced blood can no longer nourish the heart. This causes the heart to be restless and vexed, a disease called disturbance. Disturbance means a confused, vexed, oppressed, and restless heart. This is due to nonascension of the clear qi and nondescension of the turbid qi. The clear and turbid interfering with each other and being in chaos in the chest, qi and blood throughout the body counterflow and are in chaos.[2]

[2] Li Dong-yuan, *op. cit.*, p. 116

A wiry pulse as well as a rapid pulse is (due to) yin qi (*i.e.*, effulgent yin fire). When wind medicinals upbear yang to dissipate depressive fire, the rapid pulse will be mollified drastically.[3]

Anger, indignation, sorrow, worry, fear, and fright all can cause detriment to the original qi. Raging, exuberant yin fire is the result of congelation and stagnation arising in the heart and disturbances of the seven passions. The heart vessel is the abode of the spirit. When the sovereign heart is not quiet, fire is transformed. Fire is the foe to the seven spirits. Therefore, it is said that when yin fire is too effulgent, managing qi fails to enrich and nurture the spirit.[4]

The downflowing (of the five yang qi) into and their confinement with yin fire in *kun* earth is always due first to damage done by the five thieves, joy, anger, sorrow, worry, and fright, followed by stagnation of stomach qi. Finally, overtaxation and dietary irregularity succeed in damaging the original qi.[5]

Damage done by food and drink and taxation and overwork may lead to spontaneous sweating, frequent urination, yin fire overwhelming the earth phase, failure to engender the clear qi, and obstruction of the yang tract. (In that case,) fire is hidden in the yin blood.[6]

---

[3] *Ibid.*, p. 51

[4] *Ibid.*, p. 133

[5] *Ibid.*, p. 146

[6] *Ibid.*, p. 157

Hot Above, Cold Below

It is my experience that many Western patients have a combination of spleen vacuity and dampness with liver depression, qi stagnation. This may be complicated by depressive heat in the liver, stomach, lungs, and/or heart or damp heat in the lower burner. The most prominent symptoms of spleen vacuity are fatigue and loose stools. The dampness may exhibit itself as excessive phlegm, being overweight, or excessive vaginal discharge in women and turbid urine in both men and women. Typically, the tongue will be inflated and bear the indentations of the teeth on its edges. The liver depression, qi stagnation expresses itself in emotional tension, irritability, distention of the abdomen, lateral costal region, and/or breasts, flatulence, and/or menstrual irregularity in women. Depressive heat manifests itself in a bitter taste in the mouth, not just irritability but irascibility, breast pain and not just distention, inflated, possible red tongue edges, and a yellow tongue coating. If there is heat in the stomach, there may be a big appetite and acne on the areas of the face traversed by the *yang ming*. If there is heat in the lungs, there may also be acne as well as emotional lability and easy weeping. If there is heat in the heart, there may be sores on the tip of the tongue, insomnia, palpitations, and symptoms of a restless spirit.

Because of the relationship of the spleen to the blood, the spleen being the postnatal or latter heaven root of blood engenderment and transformation, spleen vacuity may easily lead to and become complicated by blood vacuity. On the other hand, depressive heat may easily transform dampness into damp heat at the same time as enduring heat damages yin, blood, and body fluids. Thus liver depression may give rise to yin vacuity symptoms. However, the spleen and kidneys also have a close mutual relationship. The spleen is the postnatal root of qi and blood transformation and engenderment, but the kidneys are the prenatal or former heaven root. Acquired essence derived from the finest essence transformed into the qi and blood by the spleen is treasured in the kidneys in order to bolster and support the prenatal or former heaven essence, while the kidneys supply the spleen with original qi for the transformation and engenderment of qi and blood. In other words, it is kidney yang which is the source and root of spleen yang. If there is enduring spleen qi vacuity, then over time and due to chronic disease or debility due to aging, spleen qi vacuity will give rise to kidney qi and eventually kidney yang vacuity.

I am a TCM gynecology specialist, so when it comes to clinical experience, I must mostly talk about female patients. In my experience, the above complicated combination of disease mechanisms is a common one in the case of Western women who are in their late 30s and early to late 40s. There may be spleen vacuity and dampness, liver depression, heat in their liver, stomach, lungs, and/or heart, possible damp heat below, liver blood vacuity, and kidney yang vacuity. In this case, the pulse is not going to be slow and deep as is the textbook norm for kidney yang vacuity and one must take great care in parsing out the various pulse images appearing in the various positions.

In this complicated pattern discrimination, there are usually large, possibly slippery, almost always floating, rootless pulses in the *cun* or inch position. Depending upon the presence of heat in the lungs or heart and the complication of blood or yin vacuity, either the right or the left *cun* may be either larger, more slippery, or floating. The *guan* or bar position will usually be wiry and fine. The left *guan* may be more wiry than the right, unless the pattern involves liver invading the stomach with upward counterflow or stomach fire, in which case, the right *guan* will frequently be more wiry, larger, and more forceful than the left. If, on the other hand, spleen vacuity and dampness are pronounced, then there may be a soggy pulse on the right *guan*, remembering that this is defined as a floating, fine, soft pulse. The cubit, foot, or *chi* positions may both be wiry if yin is not insufficient. If yin is insufficient, the left *chi* is often fine, wiry, and floating. The right *chi* may be wiry but may also be deepish, slippery, and wiry. It is also possible for both *chi* positions to be rootless or *wu gen*.

If one understands the disease mechanisms associated with each of the pulses, then this complicated pulse picture is not hard to understand. If, however, one can feel only the slippery quality of the *cun* pulses and the fact that they are large and thus thinks they are an indication of repletion, if they feel the floating quality of the *cun* positions but only remembers that the floating pulse is an indication of an exterior condition, or if they feel the slippery quality of the right *chi* and do not find out or do not take into account the symptoms of kidney yang vacuity such as the typical cold feet, nocturia, and low back and/or knee soreness and weakness, then they will not be able to understand this complicated pattern. Further, in this case, there will commonly be a light red tongue or a red tongue tip and edges. If one only feels the fine pulse at the left *chi* positions and misses that it is floating, they may see the yin and blood vacuity but also miss the yang vacuity below. Unfortunately, in my experience, such complicated patterns are the norm and not the exception in the Western practice of TCM.

Closing Advice

Therefore, my closing advice beyond memorizing the definitions of the main pulse images and understanding the mechanisms for each of these images is to keep in mind the concept of counterflow. According to Li Dong-yuan, Zhu Dan-xi, and their followers, yin fire typically results in qi surging upward or what can simply be called counterflow. This means yang qi will tend to move upward and outward in the body. This then tends to make even vacuity pulses, both yin and yang vacuity pulses, largish, slippery, and floating.

Bibliography

Chinese Language Bibliography

Mai Jing (Pulse Classic) by Wang Shu-he, Peoples' Health & Hygiene Press, Beijing, 1982

Mai Jing Xiao Shi (A School Explanation of the Pulse Classic) by Fuzhou Municipal Peoples' Hospital, Peoples' Health & Hygiene Press, Beijing, 1984

Se Mai She Zhen (Color, Pulse & Tongue Examination) by Wu Han-xiang, Shanghai Science & Technology Press, Shanghai, 1987

Yi Zong Jin Jian (Golden Mirror of Ancestral Medicine) ed. by Wu Qian, People's Health & Hygiene Press, Beijing, 1985

Zhong Guo Yi Xue Zhen Fa Da Quan (A Great, Complete [Compendium] of Methods of Medical Examination in China) by Ma Zhong-xue, Shandong Science & Technology Press, Jinan, 1991

Zhong Yi Mai Xue Ru Men (Entering the Gate of the Study of the Pulse in Chinese Medicine) by Jiang Chang-yuan, Science & Technology Literary Press, Chengdu, Sichuan, 1986

Zhong Yi Zhen Duan Xue Jie (Explanation of TCM Diagnosis) by Ji Feng-xia & Zhou Yu-long, TCM Ancient Literature Press, Beijing, 1986

Chinese-English Bibliography

Chinese-English Terminology of Traditional Chinese Medicine by Shuai Xue-zhong, Hunan Science & Technology Press, Changsha, 1983

English Language Bibliography

Chin Kuei Yao Lueh (Prescriptions from the Golden Chamber) by Zhang Zhong-jing, trans. by Wang Su-yen & Hong-yen Hsu, Oriental Healing Arts Institute, Los Angeles, CA, 1983

The Essential Book of Traditional Chinese Medicine, Vol. 1, Theory by Liu Yanchi, Columbia University Press, NY, 1988

The Essentials of Chinese Diagnostics by Manfred Porkert, Chinese Medicine Publications Inc., Zurich, Switzerland, 1983

Extra Treatises Based on Investigation & Inquiry by Zhu Dan-xi, trans. by Yang Shou-zhong & Duan Wu-jin, Blue Poppy Press, Boulder, CO, 1994

Fundamentals of Chinese Medicine, a compilation of texts from the Beijing, Nanjing, and Shanghai Colleges of TCM, trans. by Nigel Wiseman & Andy Ellis, Paradigm Publications, Brookline, MA, 1985

Glossary of Chinese Medical Terms and Acupuncture Points by Nigel Wiseman & Ken Boss, Paradigm Publications, Brookline, MA, 1990

How to Write a TCM Herbal Formula by Bob Flaws, Blue Poppy Press, Boulder, CO, 1993

Li Dong-yuan's Treatise on the Spleen & Stomach by Li Dong-yuan, trans. by Yang Shou-zhong & Li Jian-yong, Blue Poppy Press, Boulder, CO, 1993

Master Hua's Classic of the Central Viscera by Hua Tuo, trans. by Yang Shou-zhong, Blue Poppy Press, Boulder, CO, 1993

Nan Ching (The Classic of Difficult Issues), trans. by Paul U. Unschuld, University of California Press, Berkeley, CA, 1986

Pulse Diagnosis by Li Shi-zhen, trans. by Hoc Ku Hyunh, Paradigm Publications, Brookline, MA, 1981. (In actuality, this is not a translation of the *Bin Hu Mai Xue [The Lakeside Master's Study of the Pulse]* by Li Shizhen and his father but a translation of the commentary on that book appearing in *Zhong Yi Mai Xue Ru Men* cited above.)

Shang Han Lun, The Great Classic of Chinese Medicine by Zhang Zhongjing, trans. by Hong-yen Hsu & William G. Peacher, Oriental Healing Arts Institute, Los Angeles, CA, 1981

Sticking to the Point: A Rational Methodology for the Step by Step Formulation & Administration of a TCM Acupuncture Treatment by Bob Flaws, Blue Poppy Press, Boulder, CO, 2nd ed., 1994

Traditional Medicine in Contemporary China by Nathan Sivin, Center for Chinese Studies, University of Michigan, Ann Arbor, MI, 1987. This is a partial translation of *Xin Pian Zhong Yi Xue Kai Yao (Revised Outline of Chinese Medicine).*

The Web That Has No Weaver: Understanding Chinese Medicine by Ted Kaptchuk, Congdon & Weed, NY, 1983

Index

A

B

C

D

E

F

G

H

I

J, K

L

M

N, O

P

Q

R

S

T

U

V

W

X, Y

Z

OTHER BOOKS ON CHINESE MEDICINE AVAILABLE FROM BLUE POPPY PRESS

1775 Linden Ave
Boulder, CO 80304
For ordering 1-800-487-9296
PH. 303\447-8372 FAX 303\447-0740

SEVENTY ESSENTIAL TCM FORMULAS FOR BEGINNERS by Bob Flaws, ISBN 0-936185-59-7, $19.95

CHINESE PEDIATRIC MASSAGE THERAPY: A Parent's & Practitioner's Guide to the Prevention & Treatment of Childhood Illness, by Fan Ya-li, ISBN 0-936185-54-6, $12.95

RECENT TCM RESEARCH FROM CHINA, trans. by Charles Chace & Bob Flaws, ISBN 0-936185-56-2, $18.95

EXTRA TREATISES BASED ON INVESTIGATION & INQUIRY: A Translation of Zhu Dan-xi's *Ge Zhi Yu Lun*, by Yang Shou-zhong & Duan Wu-jin, ISBN 0-936185-53-8, $15.95

A NEW AMERICAN ACUPUNCTURE by Mark Seem, ISBN 0-936185-44-9, $19.95

PATH OF PREGNANCY, VOL. I, Gestational Disorders by Bob Flaws, ISBN 0-936185-39-2, $16.95

PATH OF PREGNANCY, Vol. II, A Handbook of Traditional Chinese Postpartum Diseases by Bob Flaws. ISBN 0-936185-42-2, $18.95

HOW TO WRITE A TCM HERBAL FORMULA A Logical Methodology for the Formulation & Administration of Chinese Herbal Medicine in Decoction, by Bob Flaws, ISBN 0-936185-49-X, $10.95

FULFILLING THE ESSENCE A Handbook of Traditional & Contemporary Treatments for Female Infertility, by Bob Flaws, ISBN 0-936185-48-1, $19.95

Li Dong-yuan's TREATISE ON THE SPLEEN & STOMACH, A Translation of the *Pi Wei Lun* by Yang Shou-zhong & Li Jian-yong, ISBN 0-936185-41-4, $21.95

SCATOLOGY & THE GATE OF LIFE: The Role of the Large Intestine in Immunity by Bob Flaws ISBN 0-936185-20-1 $14.95

MENOPAUSE A Second Spring: Making a Smooth Transition with Traditional Chinese Medicine by Honora Lee Wolfe ISBN 0-936185-18-X

$14.95

How to Have A HEALTHY PREGNANCY, HEALTHY BIRTH With Traditional Chinese Medicine by Honora Lee Wolfe, ISBN 0-936185-40-6, $9.95

MIGRAINES & TRADITIONAL CHINESE MEDICINE: A Layperson's Guide by Bob Flaws ISBN 0-936185-15-5 $11.95

STICKING TO THE POINT: A Rational Methodology for the Step by Step Formulation & Administration of an Acupuncture Treatment by Bob Flaws ISBN 0-936185-17-1 $14.95

ENDOMETRIOSIS, INFERTILITY AND TRADITIONAL CHINESE MEDICINE: A Laywoman's Guide by Bob Flaws ISBN 0-936185-14-7 $9.95

THE BREAST CONNECTION: A Laywoman's Guide to the Treatment of Breast Disease by Chinese Medicine by Honora Lee Wolfe ISBN 0-936185-61-9, $9.95

NINE OUNCES: A Nine Part Program For The Prevention of AIDS in HIV Positive Persons by Bob Flaws ISBN 0-936185-12-0 $9.95

THE TREATMENT OF CANCER BY INTEGRATED CHINESE-WESTERN MEDICINE by Zhang Dai-zhao, trans. by Zhang Ting-liang & Bob Flaws, ISBN 0-936185-11-2, $18.95

A HANDBOOK OF TRADITIONAL CHINESE DERMATOLOGY by Liang Jian-hui, trans. by Zhang Ting-liang & Bob Flaws, ISBN 0-936185-07-4 $15.95

A HANDBOOK OF TRADITIONAL CHINESE GYNECOLOGY by Zhejiang College of TCM, trans. by Zhang Ting-liang, ISBN 0-936185-06-6 (4nd edit.) $22.95

PRINCE WEN HUI'S COOK: Chinese Dietary Therapy by Bob Flaws & Honora Lee Wolfe, ISBN 0-912111-05-4, $12.95 (Published by Paradigm Press, Brookline, MA)

THE DAO OF INCREASING LONGEVITY AND CONSERVING ONE'S LIFE by Anna Lin & Bob Flaws, ISBN 0-936185-24-4 $16.95

FIRE IN THE VALLEY: The TCM Diagnosis and Treatment of Vaginal Diseases by Bob Flaws ISBN 0-936185-25-2 $16.95

HIGHLIGHTS OF ANCIENT ACUPUNCTURE PRESCRIPTIONS trans. by Honora Lee Wolfe & Rose Crescenz ISBN 0-936185-23-6 $14.95

ARISAL OF THE CLEAR: A Simple Guide to Healthy Eating According to Traditional Chinese Medicine by Bob Flaws, ISBN #-936185-27-9 $8.95

PEDIATRIC BRONCHITIS: Its Cause, Diagnosis & Treatment According to Traditional Chinese Medicine trans. by Gao Yu-li and Bob Flaws, ISBN 0-936185-26-0 $15.95

AIDS & ITS TREATMENT ACCORDING TO TRADITIONAL CHINESE MEDICINE by Huang Bing-shan, trans. by Fu-Di & Bob Flaws, ISBN 0-936185-28-7 $24.95

ACUTE ABDOMINAL SYNDROMES: Their Diagnosis & Treatment by Combined Chinese-Western Medicine by Alon Marcus, ISBN 0-936185-31-7 $16.95

MY SISTER, THE MOON: The Diagnosis & Treatment of Menstrual Diseases by Traditional Chinese Medicine by Bob Flaws, ISBN 0-936185-34-1, $24.95

FU QING-ZHU'S GYNECOLOGY trans. by Yang Shou-zhong and Liu Da-wei, ISBN 0-936185-35-X, $22.95

FLESHING OUT THE BONES: The Importance of Case Histories in Chinese Medicine trans. by Charles Chace. ISBN 0-936185-30-9, $18.95

CLASSICAL MOXIBUSTION SKILLS in Contemporary Clinical Practice by Sung Baek, ISBN 0-936185-16-3 $12.95

THE MEDICAL I CHING: Oracle of the Healer Within by Miki Shima, OMD, ISBN 0-936185-38-4, $19.95

MASTER TONG'S ACUPUNCTURE: An Ancient Lineage for Modern Practice, trans. and commentary by Miriam Lee, OMD, ISBN 0-936185-37-6, $19.95

A HANDBOOK OF TCM UROLOGY & MALE SEXUAL DYSFUNCTION by Anna Lin, OMD, ISBN 0-936185-36-8, $16.95

PMS: Its Cause, Diagnosis & Treatment According to Traditional Chinese Medicine by Bob Flaws ISBN 0-936185-22-8 $14.95

MASTER HUA'S CLASSIC OF THE CENTRAL VISCERA by Hua Tuo, ISBN 0-936185-43-0, $21.95

THE HEART & ESSENCE OF DAN-XI'S METHODS OF TREATMENT by Xu Dan-xi, trans. by Yang Shou-zhong, ISBN 0-926185-49-X, $21.95

STATEMENTS OF FACT IN TRADITIONAL CHINESE MEDICINE by Bob Flaws, ISBN 0-936185-52-X, $10.95

IMPERIAL SECRETS OF HEALTH & LONGEVITY by Bob Flaws, ISBN 0-936185-51-1, $9.95

THE SYSTEMATIC CLASSIC OF ACUPUNCTURE & MOXIBUSTION (*Jia Yi Jing*) by Huang-fu Mi, trans. by Yang Shou-zhong and Charles Chace, ISBN 0-936185-29-5, $79.95

CHINESE MEDICINAL WINES & ELIXIRS by Bob Flaws, ISBN 0-936185-58-9, $18.95

THE DIVINELY RESPONDING CLASSIC: A Translation of the *Shen Ying Jing* from the *Zhen Jiu Da Cheng*, trans. by Yang Shou-zhong and Liu Feng-ting ISBN 0-936185-55-4

PAO ZHI: An Introduction to Processing Chinese Medicinals to Enhance Their Therapeutic Effect, by Philippe Sionneau, ISBN 0-936185-62-1, $34.95

THE BOOK OF JOOK: Chinese Medicinal Porridges, An Alternative to the Typical Western Breakfast, by Bob Flaws, ISBN0-936185-60-0, $16.95

SHAOLIN SECRET FORMULAS for the Treatment of External Injuries, by De Chan, ISBN 0-936185-08-2, $18.95

AGING & BLOOD STASIS: A New Approach to TCM Geriatrics, by Yan De-xin, ISBN 0-936185-63-5, $21.95

CHINESE MEDICAL PALMISTRY: Your Health in Your Hand, by Zong Xiao-fan & Gary Liscum, ISBN 0-936185-64-3, $15.95

THE SECRET OF CHINESE PULSE DIAGNOSIS by Bob Flaws, ISBN 0-936185-67-8, $17.95

LOW BACK PAIN: Care & Prevention with Traditional Chinese Medicine by Douglas Frank, ISBN 0-936185-66-X, $9.95